I0455540

(More than) 50 Ways to Lose your Blubber

Written by Dave Yarnell

Certified Personal Trainer
Webmaster of Christianiron.com
Masters 2 powerlifting record holder

Table of Contents

Chapter One

Introduction

Ok, I came up with the title because it sounded catchy and maybe just a tad funny, but can I back it up??

If there are indeed 50 ways to get rid of unwanted fat on our frames, than why are so many people still overweight??

Well, maybe because there are more than 50 ways to gain our fat behinds in the present society in which most of the "fortunate" among us find ourselves.

I say fortunate, or maybe a better word is "blessed" because unlike some less fortunate folks that live in third world countries, or even in some of the economically depressed communities right here in our own country, we do not lack for much in the food department.

We have easy access to abundance and a variety of food that is un-precedented. Fast food restaurants, diners, fine dining establishments, taverns, donut shops, bakeries, grocery stores, convenience stores; the list goes on and is ever growing.

Couple that with the fact that modern technology has made previously labor-intensive chores much easier, and the fact that everything is made with reducing toil and making our lives easier in mind, and we have the double whammy that has lead to the obesity crisis in our current times.

Most people drive everywhere, even if the destination is a block or two down the road.

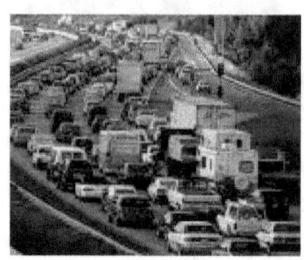

Elevators and escalators save us from the dreadful chore of actually walking up or down a flight of stairs or two.

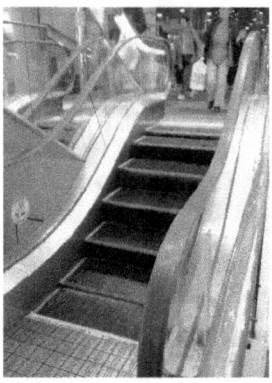

I recently watched a sitcom skit portraying a couple of people getting "stranded" on an escalator because of a short power outage.
When the escalator stopped moving, they were completely dismayed and just continued to cry out for help, rather than simply walking the remaining stairs to get to their desired level. Is this absurd? It absolutely is absurd, but how far from the truth is it, really?
I saw a picture a while back depicting a beautiful new workout facility, one of the well known names in the industry, complete with an escalator going up to the entrance!?
HELLO?!?

It is no wonder that we find ourselves shelling out big bucks to get tummy tucks, gastric bypasses, plastic surgery, etc, etc.

We are our own worst enemies, in many cases. Our children are growing up obese, too, because instead of going out with friends and playing active games and sports, they sit in front of a glowing tube that provides constant entertainment and very little else of any real value.

While they play video games or divulge personal information to complete strangers on "myspace" or something similar, they wolf down packaged, convenient snacks loaded with fat, sugar, empty calories, excessive sodium, and very little real nutrition.

Some have even charged that the food conglomerates are adding addictive substances to their foods that cause us to crave them even more, and dull our normal responses of satiation and fullness.

Even if that charge is not fully accurate, because this type of food is so devoid of real nutrition, it does leave the consumer craving more and more, without ever getting true satisfaction, which is just fine with junk food manufacturers everywhere.

Ok, so much for my rant against modern society. It still beats the heck out of trying to kill a bison with a stone-tipped spear in order to get a burger and supplementing it with some berries or perhaps a mushroom that you are not quite sure is edible, doesn't it?

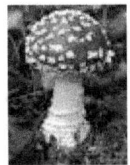

We as individuals can certainly use a bit of common sense and make the most of our modern life while still eating a reasonably sound diet and getting a little well needed exercise without making the combination unbearable. There are more "diets" out there than you can shake a carrot stick at, and unfortunately, these do more to contribute to the problem than they do to solve it, for the most part. We need to make **long-term changes** that we can stick with for life, and forget about losing massive amounts of fat in a very short time, and then returning to our old ways.

Eliminating an entire class of foods like carbohydrates or fats is unhealthy and not sustainable.

Yes, you will lose weight by doing this, at least in the short term, but eventually you will likely gain all that weight back and then some. You see it all the time with celebrities, friends; maybe even yourself.

It's time to get off of the roller coaster!

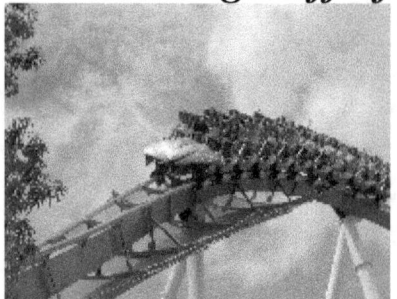

 Set some sensible, reasonable goals for the long term, and then make some shorter term goals that you can reach fairly quickly to get you in a positive frame of mind for continued success.

Losing a pound or two of fat a week is a realistic and sustainable goal, especially if you have quite a bit to lose as you start out.

When you get closer to you your "ideal" weight, it may become tougher to lose those last stubborn pounds. This is the way our bodies are designed. They prefer to keep a little something for a rainy day, so to speak. It is a design meant to stave off starvation, and it works pretty well.

Chapter Two

The List(s)

So here goes; a list of *50 legitimate ways to lose weight*!

50 ways with exercise

1) Stair climbing
2) Adding "steps"
3) Calisthenics
4) Rope jumping
5) Walking
6) Jogging
7) Running
8) Sprinting
9) Interval style Running/walking
10) Swimming
11) Biking
12) Weight training
13) Band/tube training
14) Isometrics
15) Bodyweight training
16) Playground workouts
17) Sandbag training
18) Treadmill

19) Elliptical machine
20) Stationary bike
21) Virtual resistance training
22) Iso-flexing
23) Ski motion simulators (like Nordic track, etc)
24) Aerobic dance
25) Belly dancing
26) Any type of dancing
27) Mowing the lawn
28) Shoveling snow
29) Raking leaves
30) Stationary Bike riding
31) Aerobic Stepping
32) Gardening
33) Rowing machine
34) Sculling
35) Kayaking
36) Golfing (walking from one hole to next)
37) Tennis
38) Volleyball
39) Tetherball
40) Wii fit games
41) Climbing
42) Stair climber machine
43) "Air walker"
44) Skiing
45) Snow boarding
46) Skateboarding
47) Water Skiing
48) Boxing
49) Martial arts training

50) Gymnastics

But wait! There's more!
Here are yet 50 more ways!!

50 Ways with diet

1) Replace high saturated fat food with high protein, lower fat food.
2) Add fiber to each meal
3) Replace refined sugar type snack with fruit or nuts
4) Get rid of soda and other sugary, nutrition empty drinks
5) Eat 5 or 6 smaller meals instead of 2 or 3 larger ones
6) Never eat right before bed time
7) always eat breakfast
8) read labels
9) keep a diet journal
10) eat more salads
11) skip the butter
12) try popcorn, sans butter or use low cal replacement spray, instead of chips
13) reduce sodium intake
14) drink plenty of water
15) eat a piece of fruit rather than drinking a glass of fruit juice

16) Eat yogurt regularly (try organic... the best!)
17) Top your baked potato with yogurt or salsa instead of sour cream, gravy or butter
18) Try low-fat mayo, or skip it altogether
19) Leave 25% on your plate
20) Use smaller serving plates
21) Eat smaller portions of your normal foods
22) Drink a big glass of water before each meal
23) Keep saturated fats to a bare minimum, replace with mono- unsaturated and poly-unsaturated fats
24) Cut down on creamer in your coffee or eliminate it
25) Eat more vegetables and fruits
26) Cook with extra virgin olive oil or cocoanut oil
27) Take a multi vitamin supplement
28) Replace refined white breads and pastas with whole wheat or other whole grains
29) Try yams to replace white potatoes
30) Use real honey or Stevia to replace refined sugar
31) Drop the luncheon meats, or at least opt for lower fat, lower salt varieties like lean turkey, roast beef
32) Use low fat or no-fat dairy products as opposed to regular variety
33) Try drinking some Green tea
34) Eat a grapefruit regularly
35) Keep alcohol to a modest intake
36) Have a whole wheat bagel with a dab of peanut butter instead of a couple of donuts
37) Never starve yourself!
38) Never eliminate an entire food group or class (like carbohydrates or fats)

39) Find out if you have food allergies, avoid those foods
40) Eat a little more slowly
41) Chew your food well
42) Skip dessert
43) Avoid "hydrogenated Corn Syrup"
44) Seek color in your salads… bland usually means less nutrition
45) Avoid high fat dressings on your salads
46) Avoid croutons and bacon bits on your salads
47) Try egg whites in your omelets.
48) Replace a packaged food with an organic food whenever possible and practical
49) Never eat until you are "stuffed to the gills"
50) Avoid fast food restaurants

That was easier than I thought it would be!
Well, maybe not on the diet side, but I could have easily kept going on the exercises and activities.
Really, you can break down a lot of the exercises given into more specific ones, as they are just "categories".
Under weight training alone, there could be numerous sub-headings and specific types of weight training.
You could add any number of sports activities that I did not mention.
Every day activities like carrying groceries, changing light bulbs, and so forth all burn some calories.

In fact, I recently got one of those cool watches that monitors your heart rate and tells you how many calories are burned during any specific workout or activity, and you might be surprised how many calories are burned doing some routine household chores!
I strapped on my monitor for a bout of lawn mowing with my non-motorized, dull bladed manual lawn mower, suspecting this would be a decent cardio challenge.

It really was, as I ended up burning hundreds of calories by the time I was done.

Less strenuous "sports" like bowling, throwing darts, table tennis, croquet, badminton and many more all burn some calories and could be added to the list.

What I'm getting at here is that **SOME ACTIVITY** is better than none, anyway you slice it.

Sitting completely motionless on a recliner, work chair or the sofa for countless hours, day after day will lead to poor health, a bad attitude, and extra inches in all the places we would rather not have them.

I just read an online excerpt from none other than Ben Franklin on his thoughts about fitness.

While Ben is not typically regarded as a fitness guru,

He did live to the ripe "old age" of 66 when the average lifespan for his contemporaries was more like 40 years.

So perhaps he did have some wisdom to impart in this arena, after all.

The gist of Ben's wisdom was that riding horseback was about 5 times more beneficial than riding in a horse drawn coach, walking was 5 times better than riding the horse and walking up or down stairs was 5 times better than walking on level ground.

Ben was also a pioneer of using one's heart rate to judge the quality of exercise they were doing. The higher the heart rate achieved (short of dire over-exertion), the better quality of the workout.

This has been well substantiated in our modern age, so again, Ben proved himself to be ahead of his time and no dummy!

People often will rationalize not taking any steps to getting in better shape with excuses.

"I don't like lifting weights", "I hate running", "The treadmill is boring and tedious", "Jogging is too tough on my joints", yata, yata, yata…

While lifting weights and some forms of running are well used, popular forms of getting in shape, they are *not the only ways by any means.*

Just upping your activity level, even if just a wee bit at a time, will get you on the road to fitness recovery.

Rome was not built in a day, as we have all heard before, as well as the old saying *"a journey of 1000 miles begins with one step".*

Cliché', yes, but true never the less.

While world class athletes possess incredible will power, this is not a prerequisite for simply getting in better condition. (Thank God!)

Here is a Calories burned/30 min of various activities chart that could be very helpful.
I found this at this site

http://www.recipedelights.com/calorieburning.htm

Activity (30 minutes)	Calories
Aerobic Dance	178
Basketball	258
Bicycling (10 mph, level ground)	189
Bowling (competitive)	108
Canoeing (vigorous)	192
Croquet	111
Field Hockey	249
Fishing	114
Golf (carrying clubs)	162
Golf (power cart)	108
Handball (leisure)	270
Handball (vigorous)	297
Horseback riding (galloping)	255
Horseback riding (trotting)	204
Horseback riding (walking)	75
Ice skating (fast pace)	315
Ice skating (slow pace)	199
Judo	363
Jumping rope	223
Mountain climbing	270
Rowing machine	378
Roller skating (fast pace)	315
Roller skating (slow pace)	199
Running (5.5 mph)	295
Running (7.5 mph)	426
Skiing (cross-country, 2.5 mph)	252
Skiing (cross-country, 8.0 mph)	459
Skiing (downhill)	247
Sleeping	32
Squash	393
Swimming (breast stroke, 1.0 mph)	300
Swimming (crawl, fast)	291

Swimming (back stroke)	341
Tennis (singles)	216
Tennis (doubles)	162
Volleyball	93
Walking (3.0 to 3.5 mph)	130

Keep this formula in mind:

Estimated calorie burning for common activities above is based on a 135 lb woman

10% **more** calories will be burnt for every 15 lbs over 135 lbs.

10% **less** calories will be burnt for every 15 lbs below 135 lbs.

Really, your age and general condition should also be factored in, as your resting heart rate changes along with these factors. If your resting HR is higher, you will be burning more calories, but this also means you are in poorer condition starting out.

The chart above contains some activities that I did not list in my 50, and it does not contain some of the ones I did list. I'm sure if you looked hard enough on the internet and/or in the public library, you could probably get calorie burn rate projections for just about any activity you have in mind. As I suggested earlier, you don't even have to take guesses at it.
You can strap on a heart rate monitor during any activity and get a pretty accurate actual calorie burn figure for yourself, in your present condition. Once you get a good idea of calories burned for a specific activity over a fixed period of time, you have solved one of the key equations in designing your new nutrition and activity plan.

Improvement is the key word here. *EVERYBODY* can make improvements with a little bit of honest effort.
For some that have genetic gifts, improvements may come easier, but they are not beyond anyone.
The primary reason I wanted to come up with 50 ways to exercise and lose fat, and 50 ways to make dieting changes to lose fat, is to show everyone

that there are a heck of a lot of ways to "skin a cat" (That doesn't mean what you think, PETA people)

I really feel that *if you take a good look at both of the lists given above, you will find at least a few ideas that you can incorporate into your lifestyle without feeling beaten up, deprived or tortured.*

One of the *"bad words" in the exercise world is "routine"*

Too many exercise programs become exactly that, in a very short time, and it is probably *boredom* that *puts more fitness plans to rest than injuries or other issues.*

Besides, "*going through the motions*" of an exercise scheme without enjoying it or really having your heart in it will be far less fruitful than if you look forward to each workout with zeal. Some folks are able to "*get in the zone*"; even doing the same types of workouts continuously for long stretches. These are the folks that are more prone to becoming superior athletes, world class bodybuilders, weightlifters, etc.

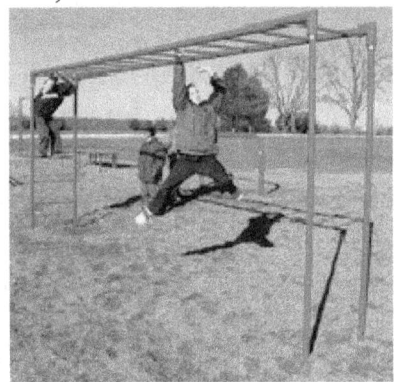

And then there are the rest of us.

Most of us were more active as children, getting plenty of exercise without considering it boring or the least bit tedious. We were simply playing and having fun.

We played games of pick-up ball of all kinds, maybe jumped some rope, played hop-scotch, games involving running after each other, throwing balls, Frisbees, and on and on.

Did we get home at the end of one of these glorious days and say "man that was a killer workout?"

Not likely, I'd say.

As we got older, many of us got chained to a desk or perhaps some other sedentary form of making a living.

We "put away childish things", which is great in some ways, but it did have some *negative consequences.*

Lots of folks played sports while in high school, perhaps into the college years, but usually by the early to mid twenties, these activities were at least greatly curtailed, if not completely abandoned.

I was taught to "*clean my plate*" at dinner, or I could not have ice cream or some other delicacy afterwards.

I'm sure many of you that are anywhere near my age and even some who are not will have had similar experiences.

When we lead the active lifestyles that most of us did (at least relative to our current ones), we could eat like horses and never get "fat".

Of course, hormones certainly played a role in that also.

As a society, we have allowed ourselves to think that it is completely normal and natural to gain inches around the middle and elsewhere, get weaker, less energetic and develop more aches and pains as we grow older.

Just the fact that this does indeed happen in most cases seems to be enough evidence for us to buy into the whole concept, hook, line and sinker.

The question we should be asking is this: *do we slow down our activity levels, ability to perform and be energetic because of our getting older, or is it at least partially the other way around?*

Do we get older, weaker, fatter and less energetic *BECAUSE* we slowed down our activity/exercise level??

It is very easy to look around and find people who have somehow managed to defy the ageing process, at least to some degree.

We could point to Jack Lalanne, who as of this writing is 94 and still going strong. Jack has said that inactivity causes aging more than anything, with perhaps the exception of a poor diet.

We can write this off (longevity) to good genes, better environment, etc., but I think we are kidding ourselves if we think these are the real primary factors. Sure, genetics plays a role in health and longevity, no doubt. Ask any person who has reached the age of 100 or more, what the secret of their longevity and health is and you will find a *common thread* in all or most. That common thread is *remaining active.*

I am not suggesting that 100 year olds are running marathons, entering the Worlds Strongest Man contest, or pumping iron with Arnold and friends.

They may simply do some gardening on a regular basis, walk the dog around the block once or twice a week, continue to carry their own groceries, or other simple things like these. It is a well known fact that many people pass away within a couple of years of retiring.

They have been looking forward for their whole adult lives to the time when they **can stop working and do nothing at all.**

The grim reaper smiles whenever that thought crosses the soon to be retired person's gray matter.

It is the **kiss of death**! *We were designed to keep moving through our entire lives, not become sedentary at middle age, or at any specific time after that.*

When muscles are not being used on a regular basis, what happens?

They shrink and become less flexible, that's what happens. It's the old *"use it or lose it"* concept.

If you are not a weightlifter, football player, bodybuilder or strength athlete you may think "big deal", what do I need a lot of muscle for? So what if I lose some?

Besides the obvious implications of being generally weaker, there are other concerns.

Muscle **burns fuel** (fat, calories in general) much more efficiently than non-muscle tissue, so now our metabolism has been slowed down.

Add that to the **already slowed metabolism** that comes with lower hormone levels associated with getting older.

Now factor in the fact that we are probably *still eating the same or more calories than we did when our metabolism was racing, and it becomes fairly a no-brainer to see how we've come into the poor condition that we have.*

Eugen Sandow, the great strongman of old said that if we lead the lives of children or "savages", there would be no real need for "exercise routines". We would get all the needed exercise in our daily routines without ever having given it a second thought.

One of the negative consequences of our becoming more civilized is that we have become less active and more sedentary in the process.

Manual labor is avoided in most cases like the plague, yet its avoidance has caused a plague of its own, in many respects. Machines do much of our work for us, and we seek convenience rather than effort in everything we do.

We rely on elevators, escalators, driving our cars everywhere, (including a block down the road), etc, etc. I do not propose that we step back in time and give up all of our modern conveniences, but **we do need some exercise and activity in our lives.**

Chapter Three

Changing our bad eating habits

Another negative aspect of "modern society" is "convenience foods" and "fast foods".

This is another big factor in the "fattening up" of our society lately.

I am not one of these guys that are going to tell you that every food you find in a box or package is going to kill you, or that the government and the big food and drug manufacturers are running some kind of elaborate conspiracy to keep you sick and addicted.

With that being said, There are some downsides to all this.

The big food manufacturers are out to make money, like any other business is. They are **well aware of the popular trends in dieting**, etc.

When the trend in "fitness wisdom" is low fat, they will provide food with that in mind, with that magic ingredient or lack thereof prominently displayed on the front of the package.

What they are not going to display on the front of the package is that they have replaced the fat with sugar, or even worse, "high fructose corn syrup", trans fats or other unhealthy ingredients.

This is why I suggest that you learn to **read labels** on a regular basis.

Striving for better **quality** food as opposed to just reducing the **quantity** of food will go a long way towards getting and **keeping** you in good shape.

Skipping meals or eliminating entire food classes is just not going to work for the **long term.**

You may ask: isn't a calorie a calorie regardless of its origin?

To that question I would answer "yes and no".

For example, your body actually **burns calories at varying levels during the digestion of food.** Protein rich foods require more energy to process, generally speaking, as do foods with more fiber content.

Refined sugar and white bread require much less energy to process, and cause the undesirable insulin spike that causes a host of problems.

This is why eating more organic, unrefined foods is superior.

While the calories in the unrefined product may be similar in number to its refined counterpart for a given meal, you will get more nutrition out of it, with less of an insulin spike, and you get the added bonus that your body works harder to digest and process it.

Replace a candy bar with a piece of fruit or a serving of nuts. "*Go organic*" with the items you can afford to and have reasonable access to.

Use "*whole foods*" instead of refined foods whenever possible. *Whole grains* are always more nutritious and healthier than refined "white" versions that have been stripped of much of the good stuff God put in the original versions.

They have *more fiber* in them, which helps in good digestion and keeps the digestive system running more smoothly and regularly.

Fiber also gives more "*bulk*" to foods, which makes you feel fuller faster.

Of course, there are those who have *Gluten allergies* and need to stay away from even wheat, along with all the breads and related products that typically contain Gluten.

(We will discuss some alternative grains further along, by the way).

Just because you do not have an immediate, large reaction to Gluten, or anything else, does not always mean you do not have an allergy to it.

Food allergies are one of the areas that can cause people much difficulty in their weight-loss efforts, among other things.

Use honey or Stevia instead of refined white sugar or other, not-so–healthy sugar substitutes.

Many studies have shown that artificial sweeteners can be addictive and cause health concerns.

Do not assume that because a soda or other soft drink says

"diet" on the label that it can or should be consumed indiscriminately.

Water is suggested by most nutrition experts, diet book writers and doctors as something that should be consumed in large quantities, especially by those seeking to lose weight.

Every soda you drink, though it does contain some water, is displacing a certain amount of water you might otherwise drink in its place.

Drinking soda can actually deplete calcium from your bones and therefore can contribute to osteoporosis, as well as having other deleterious effects.

Drinking water is another thing that *aids in the removal of waste products in a timely fashion, and in flushing toxins out of the system.*

The body is composed largely of water, so it only stands to reason that we need to drink lots of it daily.

Having a nice tall glass of water before eating a meal will make you feel fuller and you will therefore be likely to eat less at the meal.

Taking a couple of fiber chews or something like this along with the water will enhance the filling effects.

I recently saw an ad on the tube for a new diet based on exactly this; drinking a tall glass of water laced with extra fiber before each meal.

I'm sure it is at least somewhat effective, but there is no need to purchase a special regimen or plan to carry this out on your own.

Fruits and vegetables, the fresher the better, are great for you and few of us eat enough of these on a regular basis.

What passes for a salad for many of us is simply some iceberg lettuce with some croutons, bacon bits and a big glob of fatty dressing.

This is not a real salad!

Go for the **darker green and purple/green lettuces**, spinach leaves, dandelions and sprouts to compose the green base of your salad.

Add **lots of colors**, with beets, carrots, squashes, olives, Broccoli, seeds, beans of all kinds, and any other fresh veggies and fruits you like.

Add a little protein in the form of some lean turkey, roast beef, tuna (easy on the mayo!), or some egg whites, and you have a salad that is fit for a good meal, all by itself.

Use a light vinaigrette or other low-fat dressing and skip the croutons, bacon bits and such other fatty additions.

Throw in some seeds or nuts for the crunchiness as well as the added nutrition.

In the following photo I show my typical workday lunch.
It's a little bit different every day, but always full of color and nutrition.
Try something new in your salad on a regular basis, you may find something you really enjoy and that is great for you, too!

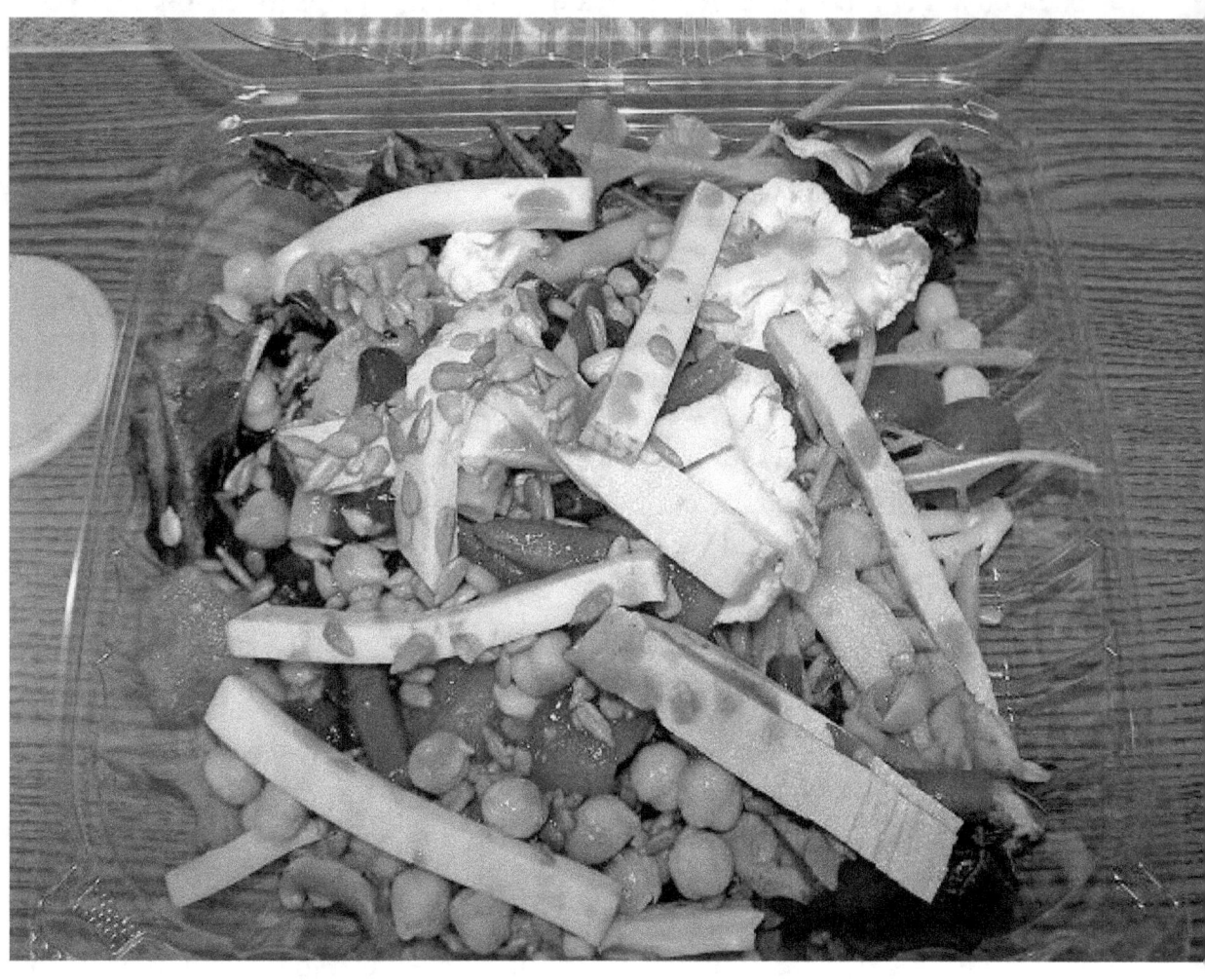

Stay away from fried foods of all kinds, and opt instead for baked, broiled or grilled as often as possible.

A piece of grilled or broiled chicken breast, sans breading, is far superior nutritionally to a fried, breaded piece.

The same holds true for fish and pork items, obviously.

Deli meats, sausages, hot-dogs and the like should not be consumed on a regular basis as they contain lots of fat, nitrites and nitrates and are generally high in sodium and/or MSG. (monosodium Glutamate)

Summer barbecues can be problematic, as hot dogs, sausages and full fat burgers are the norm at many of these events. Opt for chicken from the grill if it is available, and discard the skin to get rid of a lot of the fat based calories. A basic beef burger, when cooked on the grill, will be superior to the tube steak in terms of more nutrition and less additives.

You can even grill veggies, and use whole wheat rolls to make the offerings a little healthier.

A hot dog or bratwurst here and there over the course of a summer won't kill you; just try not to make a regular habit of it.

Turkey and lean roast beef from the deli, as well as real chicken slices are better choices for making sandwiches if you insist on buying meats from the deli section of the grocery store. They also have low-fat, low sodium varieties of the above, which are better for you.

Eating **higher quality** foods will reduce all kinds of diet related problems.

Blood sugar will not fluctuate as wildly.

Blood pressure levels will also improve in many cases.

Cholesterol levels and other lipids profiles will improve.

Internal inflammation will be far less of a problem.

Digestion will greatly improve and gastro-intestinal problems will lessen or go away all together.

The bottom line is that you will feel much better and be much healthier.

You don't have to become some kind of "health food nut".

You don't have to become a scientist or nutritionist either.

Here is a little list I put together called "America's 10 most unwanted"

America's 10 most unwanted: Wanted: dead and gone!

1. white sugar, white bread, white rice, "wheat" flour products (Not Whole wheat)

2. trans fats

3. "hydrogenated" anything

4. soda

5. High Fructose Corn Syrup

6. High Glycemic index, low nutrition value Carbohydrates

7. "Low Carb" diets

8. Excessive Alcohol consumption

9. Ingestion/absorption of toxins

10. Sedentary lifestyle

What are the problems with some of these ingredients?

High Fructose Corn Syrup, affectionately known as HFCS

This ugly but very common ingredient is a sort of "*super sugar*" that will spike insulin levels and is even worse than refined white sugar.
It can be found in yogurts (rendering an *otherwise healthy food* not so great anymore).
Oddly enough, it is often found in "nutrition bars", "diet" drinks and many items that proudly claim to be "low fat".
Being low in fat is great, but when you add in the HFCS, much of the benefit is lost, if not all of it.
One other problem with this ingredient is that *it may turn off your hunger signal feedback system.*
You may actually feel hungrier after eating a snack or beverage laden with this stuff!
This is one property that has caused some to claim that the food industry is trying to "hook" you and make you fat.
I think it is probably more about economics, in reality.
This is a man-made substitute for sugar that's whole purpose was to make the product *cheaper to manufacture.*
Fructose has some issues when compared with glucose, though it sometimes gets a pass because it is called "fruit sugar".

According to Jordan Rubin, author of "*Perfect Weight America*" and "*The Maker's Diet*", the body metabolizes fructose into triglycerides (the body's fat storage form) more than other sugars.
It also raises the risk of heart disease, and fails to stimulate the hormone that tells us we are full (Leptin), like other sugars, according to Rubin.
The liver has trouble metabolizing it, to boot.
Sodas and other sweet soft drinks are the biggest culprits, and are where about 2/3 of American's intake of this vile stuff (High Fructose Corn Syrup)come from.
If you see this ingredient on the label, it is best a product to be avoided.

Another man-made ingredient is *Trans fats*

What are the downsides to this little gem?

The latest trend is packaging with the proclamation

"low in trans fats" or "zero trans fats" on the front of the package. That is because they have been bad-mouthed by nutrition experts in a big-time way lately, as they deserve to be. Trans fats are made by heating liquid vegetable oils with hydrogen present to make them solid at room temperature.

This is called *hydrogenation. Keep that word in mind!*

Anytime you see hydrogenated…. anything, beware!

Once again, this is done for cost effective manufacture, with little regard for the health risks to the consumer.

Margarine is one of the items frequently found to contain this, but it is in many "convenience foods" from frozen pizza to salad dressing.

Europeans were ahead of the curve on this one, strictly limiting their use since 2004.

Another thing to be concerned about is the loopholes that let manufacturers put Trans fats in their products yet claim them to be "trans-fat free"

This is allowed if there are less than 500mg PER SERVING of the nasty ingredient in the product.

This is yet another reason why you MUST learn to read labels and avoid these horrible things as much as possible!

Refined foods

What's the big deal with *refined products* like white bread, white sugar, etc? Well, the big problem with these is that they have been largely *stripped of their nutrients.*

They contain less fiber and bulk, along with vitamins and minerals, etc.

Now, you might say; the package says "*vitamin enriched*",

So doesn't that make up for the losses?

NO, it does not.

Throwing a few vitamins in will not come close to replacing all that was lost in the processing.

The lost bulk and fiber also means that the carbohydrates in the bread or other product will be absorbed and turned to simple sugar much more quickly than in the whole grain product. This *spikes insulin levels and causes havoc with blood sugar levels*, as well as putting extra burdens on the liver and digestive systems.

Pasta gets a bad rap because of its relatively high glycemic index. Opt for whole wheat varieties for a better choice.

Brown or wild rice is superior to white rice, also.

The bottom line is the less processed and refined, the better the quality of the product, in general.

It's hard to improve on God's diet plan.

Some other healthy choices of complex carbohydrates are readily available also.

The following section will alternatives:

Less Common Types of Whole Grains

While we are on the topic of whole foods versus refined foods, I thought we should discuss some alternative whole grains. Some of these may be very familiar to you, but others may be new to you.

The most common types of whole grains are whole wheat, brown rice, oats, popcorn, barley, and wild rice. Less common types of whole grains include:

Amaranth:

This is a golden colored grain with a nutty flavor and a chewy texture. It can be added to flour or to thicken sauces, or used in cereals or in the same way you would use rice. This grain contains good levels of protein, iron and calcium along with its complex carbohydrates. Amaranth seed is high in protein (15-18%) and contains respectable amounts of lysine and methionine, two essential amino acids that are not frequently found in grains. It is high in fiber and contains calcium, iron, potassium, phosphorus, and vitamins A and C.

The fiber content of amaranth is three times that of wheat and its iron content, five times more than wheat. It contains two times more calcium than milk. Using amaranth in combination with wheat, corn or brown rice results in a complete protein as high in food value as fish, red meat or poultry is.

Amaranth also contains tocotrienols (a form of vitamin E) which have cholesterol-lowering activity in humans. Cooked amaranth is 90% digestible and because of this ease of digestion, it has traditionally been given to those recovering from an illness or ending a fasting period. Amaranth consists of 6-10% oil, which is found mostly within the germ. The oil is predominantly unsaturated and is high in linoleic acid, which is important in human nutrition.

The amaranth seeds have a unique quality in that the nutrients are concentrated in a natural "nutrient ring" that surrounds the center, which is the starch section. For this reason the nutrients are protected during processing. The amaranth leaf is nutritious as well containing higher calcium, iron, and phosphorus levels than spinach. It does not contain gluten, Therefore it makes a great substitute grain for those with gluten allergies or sensitivity.

Some of the info above was taken from:

http://www.chetday.com/amaranth.html

Farro:

Another grain with a nutty flavor and it can be bought in flour form to make pasta or baked goods. In its natural state, it needs lots of cooking time to tenderize, but its loaded with protein, fiber and vitamins, as well as magnesium. This ad copy from an online health food purveyor describes it as follows:

Farro is literally the first grain - the grain from which all grains have descended. *Tritucum dicoccum* has been growing in the Mediterranean for thousands of years and only dwindled in popularity due to its difficulty to grow and harvest. Farro is an unhybridized, or pure form of wheat with the husk intact. It's nutty flavor and firm, chewy texture make it versatile to no end. It plays very well with other fruits of the earth like legumes and leafy vegetables. Since the outer husk adheres to the grain, the fiber & Vitamin E content is very high. While we'd never forego taste for healthfulness, if we can find both in one place, you can count us in!

The food world has really been buzzing lately about farro; its health properties, its wonderful flavor, its texture. But a line seems to have been drawn in the sand regarding pearled or semi-pearled farro. **For the record, Rustichella d'Abruzzo's whole farro is semi-pearled and that's the way we like it.** While the pearled is easier and quicker to cook, the nutrients vanish with the husk, along with a good bit of the flavor.

See:
http://markethallfoods.com/store/index.php?main_page=product_mh_info&cPath=11_28&products_id=92&gclid=COfg3d2wgpsCFc0B4wodqh5yrw

Millet:

This is a very small grain that also can be used like rice or mixed with vegetables and fruits, or to make breads, muffins and other baked goods. The minerals in this are manganese, magnesium and phosphorous, in addition to its protein and carbohydrates. **Millet is highly nutritious, non-glutinous and like buckwheat and quinoa, is not an acid forming food so is soothing and easy to digest.** In fact, it is considered to be one of the least allergenic and most digestible grains available and it is a warming grain so will help to heat the body in cold or rainy seasons and climates.

Millet is tasty, with a mildly sweet, nut-like flavor and contains a myriad of beneficial nutrients. It is nearly 15% protein, contains high amounts of fiber, B-complex vitamins including niacin, thiamin, and riboflavin, the essential amino acid methionine, lecithin, and some vitamin E. It is particularly high in the minerals iron, magnesium, phosphorous, and potassium.

The seeds are also rich in phytochemicals, including Phytic acid, which is believed to lower cholesterol, and Phytate, which is associated with reduced cancer risk.

See: http://www.chetday.com/millet.html for more info

Triticale

 A type of whole grain that is a hybrid of rye and wheat, triticale has a nutty-rye flavor and can be used in preparing baked goods such as breads and muffins. Triticale is a good source of protein, manganese magnesium and folate.

You can find out a lot more Here:

http://www.hort.purdue.edu/newcrop/afcm/triticale.html

Spelt

Another name for Farro, this is a mineral rich grain that is available in flour or whole grain form, with a nutty taste like some of the others mentioned. You can also buy packaged spelt breads and pastas if you are not a do it yourselfer. This grain also contains manganese, protein, niacin and phosphorous.

Buying and Storing Bulk Whole Grains

These grains are becoming available more widely now, but health food and specialty stores may be your best bet at a variety of these products.

They need to be stored in airtight containers and refrigerated if bought in bulk. You might want to try a small amount first to make sure you like it.

Low "carb" diets

The Atkins diet, south beach diet and some other popular diets propose extreme limitations on carbohydrate intake in order to lose weight.

The underlying concept is to purposely trick the body into burning body fat as an **energy source** by depriving it of its normal, favored energy source… carbohydrates.

Does it work? Yes, it will cause weight loss, at least in the short term. The diet became popular in part because meat lovers could still eat steak, and other fatty foods could be consumed at will.

This diet is **not healthy or sustainable in the long term.**

Most folks who lost weight on this program gained it back when their inevitable "carb" cravings kicked in with a vengeance.

Besides that, restricting carbohydrates drastically can cause serious blood sugar issues, and has even been implicated in pre-diabetes and adult onset diabetes diagnoses.

In the same way, restricting fats to almost zilch is not a good idea in the long run either. The body needs fats, carbohydrates and proteins in their correct ratios to thrive. The body actually makes hormones using cholesterol, for example.

Manipulating hormones and weight loss by restricting any one of these may help you reach short term goals, but is almost sure to bite you in the backside in the longer term!

It makes much more sense to **reduce overall caloric intake,** and reduce (not eliminate) "bad fats" but not overly restrict the good ones.

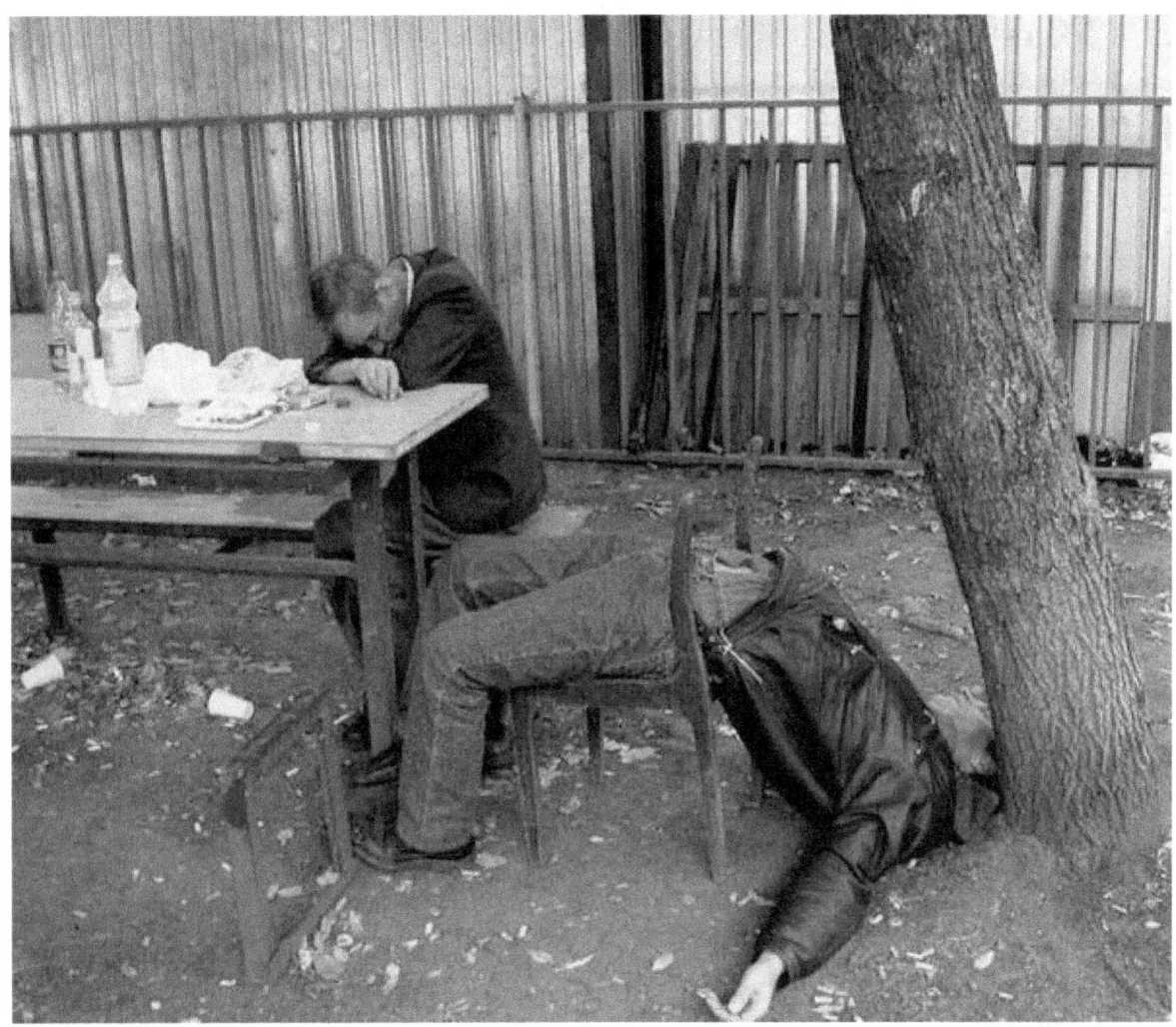

Excessive drinking

What is considered too much? For some people, 1 drink is too much.
Alcohol can be as addictive as any hard drug, especially if one has such a
predisposition.
If someone in your family is or was an alcoholic, it may suggest that it's in
your genes for you to go that route also.
Many folks are proud that they can indeed "hold their liquor", but at what
long-term cost?

For most people, a glass or two of wine or one or two beers or the equivalent is OK to consume, and some may even say there are some benefits involved. **Resveretrol** is one of the anti-oxidants that are all the rage lately, and it is found in red wine.

Many health benefits have been associated with the **moderate** use of wine, but drinking a bottle every night is going to not only cancel any potential benefits, it is almost certain to cause long-term health issues, not the least of which has to do with the **massive amount of calories** ingested.

If you are trying to lose weight (if you're reading this, you most likely are), then the extra calories of even a couple of drinks a day may not be worth it. The average 12 ounce beer contains about 150 calories, while a typical shot of whiskey is about half of that.

Typical white and red wines are around 60-80 calories per typical serving, but Sweet vermouth has almost twice that.

As you can see, if you were to drink a 6 pack of regular beer, you would be consuming almost 1000 calories.

Throw in some salty chips, nuts, pretzels or other snacks that are typically consumed along with the beers and you have really gone off the reservation! And keep in mind that higher alcohol content, micro brewery style beers are typically even higher in calories.

There are other ways to "unwind" before bed or after a hard day at the office. One alternative is the popular over the counter supplement **Melatonin.**

This is something that everyone normally has in their bodies, but it diminishes with age. Melatonin is one of the key reasons that a baby "**sleeps like a baby**", and it can help you do the same.

Besides the great calming effect, it has also been reported to enhance the normal spike in HGH (Human Growth Hormone), associated with sleep. HGH, among other things, burns fat, so it is a great alternative calming agent for those trying to trim down, and is easy to obtain, safe to use and inexpensive.

This hormone also helps to build muscle and connective tissues as well. Herbal teas like chamomile and some others are also good alternatives, as long as you go easy on the sugar or sugar substitute additives involved.

Another supplement that works well for this is the amino acid L-Tryptophan, which was banned from the market for a while because there was some tainted product that did some serious harm a few years back.

I had taken this product prior to the ban, and it was a great natural sleep aid, as well as having the same reported benefits of increasing normal HGH output as Melatonin does. The ban has been lifted on this product now.

Toxins

There are many toxins besides the obvious ones like excessive alcohol and tobacco so common in our society.

Fish can contain **Mercury and PCB's**. Common cleaning products, pesticides and other household things can be loaded with nasty ingredients. Our workplaces often expose us to a host of questionable chemicals, etc. Old houses and other buildings may expose us to **asbestos, lead paint,** and other dangerous things.

The liver and kidneys get a major workout trying to rid the blood of such invaders. Exposing ourselves knowingly to excessive amounts of alcohol and other toxins just does not make much sense.

Even Tylenol and other such over-the counter pain relievers can be toxic if over-done.

There is a trend toward "green" products for cleaning the home, killing pests, etc, and these are often very good alternatives with far less potential for toxic interactions.

You may want to try some of these and see how they work for you.

Sedentary Lifestyle

We talked about this earlier in the book, but it bears repeating.
You burn no calories (or at least very few) sitting and lying around doing nothing.
We discussed lots of ways to "get it in gear", and it is really important that you make an effort to try one or two or more of these. If you can find a calorie burning activity that you really enjoy, you will be working towards a happier, healthier, more productive lifestyle for the rest of your life.
This is not just about extending your lifespan, but about adding *quality* to your life.

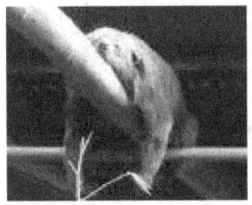

Chapter Four

Other helpful ideas

What else can we do too get in better shape?

There are a vast variety of potions, powders and pills that folks have claimed can get you in the best shape of your life. Do they work?

Some do, at least to some extent, but some not so much.

Beware of "fat burning formulas" that are loaded with **over the counter stimulants** as the primary ingredient.

Stimulants used sparingly and in the right circumstances are not all bad. You may enjoy a cup of coffee before a workout, which is not really a horrible thing. Caffeine is said to have "thermogenic" effects. (fat burning)

The now popular energy drinks contain large amounts of caffeine and **huge amounts of sugar**, so you may be better off with that cup of coffee.

Keep the added sugar to a minimum, as well as cream.

Herbal formulas have been used by many for a long time, and some have value. There are even many herbs that are commonly used in cooking that have powers that often get lost in the shuffle these days.

Consider that many drugs are actually derived from herbs.

The drugs tend to concentrate the main active ingredients of certain herbs and are usually more potent than their herbal alternatives, which has its pros and cons.

Herbs have a "gentler" interaction with the body than drugs do and may take longer to produce results, but for the same reasons are safer and have far less side effects.

This book is not intended to be an herbal book, but I will mention a few herbs that may be worthy of trying for some of you.

Garlic

Here is a very common herb that is added to foods regularly. While it is vilified for its stench, it should not be avoided because of it.

You can get odor-free garlic supplements if you don't like putting it in your food, or don't get enough that way.

Garlic is in the same family as onions and contains anti-oxidants, reduces the incidence of certain cancers, lowers bad cholesterol and high blood pressure, and has even been reported to *boost testosterone levels* and help with fat-loss.

Hoodia

This herb has been popular of late for its reported appetite suppressing qualities. The story is that native peoples have used it when going on long treks where food might be scarce.

I have no personal experience with this herb, but have read some positive reports on it, and it may be worth a try.

According to things I have read and heard, this herb is *not a thermogenic aid* (does not speed up your metabolism), but it does have some appetite suppressing qualities.

Adaptogenic herbs

These herbs are not directly associated with weight loss in general but they can help through indirect means.

Adaptogenic means they help you adapt. Adapt to what?

The answer is stress, of various types.

While this is not an all-encompassing list, here are several of these types of herbs:

Ginseng

*Licorice (*not the candy)

Ashwagandha

Rhodiola

Of the above, you may only be familiar with the more commonly known Ginseng.

Ginseng has been used for thousands of years and has been claimed to do lots of great things.

I use it myself, and I think it helps lessen the frequency and severity of colds and viruses as well as just a generally enhanced attitude and sense of well-being.

It has been suggested that it boosts immune function.

Ginseng has also been claimed to be an aphrodisiac.

Sea Kelp

While not technically an herb, but more of a food, this is the only natural substance I could find proclaimed as useful and effective as a *"reducing aid"* in a dated version of a non-prescription drug reference manual.

It is often used as a food additive. *It absorbs water* therefore can create a "filling wad" in the stomach, making one feel fuller, thus leading to les over-all calories consumed at a given meal.

Other such substances have been used in various weight loss formulas, such as Psyllium, Chondrus, Guar gum, Xanthan gum and some others.

These all can add fiber to a meal, which not only makes you feel fuller, but can soften the insulin spike of an otherwise high glycemic index food, as previously mentioned.

You may find some of these items listed on the ingredient labels of your favorite "diet" foods.

Some newer (not really new but more recently becoming popular) fiber choices that may be superior to the previous list, are *glucomannan and konjac.*

(Konjac actually contains glucomannan).

According to author and doctor Mark Hyman (*Ultrametabolism*), these substances have been connected with lowering cholesterol and inflammation (one of the underlying causes of difficult weight reduction issues).

The Ultrametabolism book goes on to list a number of other herbs that are reported to fight inflammation, as follows:

Capsaicin (from Cayenne pepper)
Green Tea
Ginger
Quercitin
Turmeric
Cocoa (yes, that's right!)

Of the items listed above, Green tea is one of the popular diet aid ingredients these days, and it is probably at least somewhat living up to the hype. Some of the rest will not be as familiar.

Ok, you have seen me make several references now to *inflammation.* When we typically think of inflammation, we may think of something being inflamed on the external part of the body, or a muscle being inflamed after an injury.
The inflammation I speak of here is of the internal variety.
Going back to Dr. Hyman, the book *Ultrametabolism* has an entire chapter devoted to inflammation, why it is so bad, and what can be done about it.
The book makes references to recent research that has suggested that obesity and inflammation are linked.
There is a vicious circle wherein being overweight causes inflammation, and inflammation causes people to be overweight.
The normal symptoms of inflammation are pain, redness, swelling and heat.
It is a part of the *body's defense system against invasions, irritation, foreign matter, etc.*
In a perfectly healthy person, there is a balance going on where there is JUST ENOUGH inflammation to keep these invaders from doing their worst.
Sometimes, this natural balance goes haywire and *inflammation runs rampant*, causing more problems than it solves.
Inflammation in different areas of the body can cause different problems.
Arthritis is an inflammatory disease and research has now been suggesting it (inflammation) as a cause of heart disease, dementia, diabetes and various other issues associated with aging.
According to *Ultrametabolism*, again, the most common cause of inflammation in our society today is related to our horrible diets.

Refined sugars, excessive animal fat intake, processed foods in general, and foods with high glycemic loads (ever so popular in the typical American diet) all contribute to inflammation.

Other contributors are stress, toxins, infections and allergens, along with *lack of exercise.*

Armed with this information, we would do well to adjust our lifestyles and diets to keep inflammation to a minimum, and adding some of the above-listed herbs to your diet may be one easy way to start to get a handle on this problem.

Inflammation is also a common theme in the book "*Perfect Weight America*", by Jordan Rubin, and "*Nutrition and Diet Therapy*", by Ruth Roth and Carolyn Townsend.

Kevin Trudeau mentions it in his books, and other prominent nutritionists and authors on the subject also bring up the subject of inflammation, so this is a *common theme* and one that should not be ignored or over-looked by the person trying to get to their ideal weight.

Chapter Five

More beneficial herbs and natural substances

Going back to something we mentioned above, there are many forms of supplemental **glucomannan** around these days and there have been studies suggesting it has value for the health and in helping aid weight loss.
Another nutrition and diet "guru", Andrew Weil has been suggesting eating the Asian noodles that contain this fiber as possibly a better alternative to the various supplements.
A couple of traditional Japanese dishes he mentioned are
Shirataki noodles (or konnyaku).

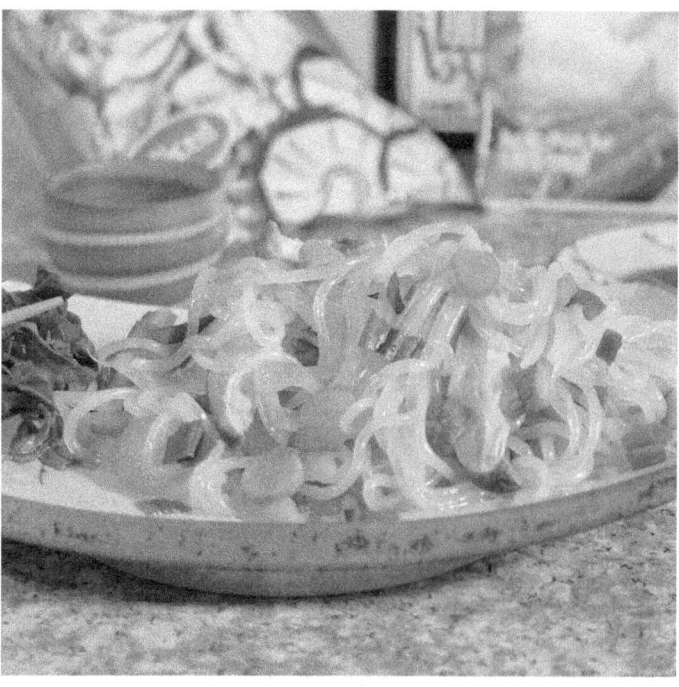

According to the Asianfoodgocer.com,
Shirataki Noodles are **the famed miracle noodle seen in several health magazines available now at Asian Food Grocer. These low- carb noodles satisfy your spaghetti cravings, and are a gluten free replacement for pasta. Shirataki Noodles are made from yams, and are naturally low in calories and carbs, plus they are an excellent source of fiber, depending on the brand you prefer. These low fat noodles are tender and absorb the flavors you cook them with, so be creative and try them with every meal. If you are a health-conscious eater then Shirataki Noodles are for you:**

More herbs

According to "***The Herb Bible***", (Paragon Publishing),
Comfrey is yet another anti-inflammatory herb.
This book also mentions "*Cleansing herbs*" that help detoxify the body, such as *elder and peppermint*.
Other anti-inflammatory herbs mentioned in this book are *calendula and aloe vera.*
Aloe is often found in gels and lotions to soothe the pain from burns, rashes, etc. In fact, I just used one of these on a sunburned area this morning and found it quite refreshing.
Two more herbs are noted as Diuretics; *dandelion and nettle.* A diuretic is something that causes excretion of water from the body, either in the form of urine or sweat.
These might be used in the process of a natural "cleanse", but should not be used to promote weight loss for extended periods of time.
Echinacea and red clover are mentioned as immune supporters, useful in detoxifying the blood and renewing tissue, according to the authors.
Horsetail and yarrow are also named as diuretics, and borage and celery are reported to be adrenal tonics, useful as pick-me-ups.
Both g*inseng and ginger* are said to be tonics for the male sex organs.

These herbs are mentioned as natural stimulant alternatives; *rosemary and peppermint.*

Another popular supplement these days is **Omega 3's, Omega-6's**, and/or fish-oil capsules.

Fish oil capsules contain lots of Omega-3's.

According to Mauro DiPasquale, a former world-class powerlifter and another expert on nutrition, our diets tend to be lop-sided towards getting more Omega-6's than we might really need, but **not enough Omega-3's.**

Eating fish that are rich in Omega 3's is OK, but eating too much of these fish could cause an intake of too much mercury and PCB's, which is certainly not what we want.

Salmon is one of these fish, and wild salmon are preferable to farm raised salmon, as they have more nutrients and less toxins.

It is suggested that if you use fish-oil capsules to get your Omega-3's, it is better to get the highest quality, **pharmaceutical grade** of these capsules to avoid the potential toxins.

These **essential fatty acids** are what could be referred to as beneficial fats. They aid in the metabolism of other dietary fats, and are essential to other critical bodily functions.

Yet another "friendly fat" is **CLA, or conjugated linoleic acid.** This stuff has been reported to **reduce body fat while preserving muscle tissue.**

CLA is found in some of the new fat loss formulas and is a healthy and promising alternative to over the counter stimulant based products.

Virgin Cocoanut Oil

Is there such a thing as a good saturated fat?

Yes, oddly enough, there actually are some relatively "good" saturated fats. As bad a rap as the group has in general, and rightfully so, they are not all equally horrible.

After all, the brain is made of about 60 percent fats, including the omega 3's we previously mentioned, and another good one called lauric acid.

The human mammary glands actually produce a fair amount of saturated fat, which is needed for early growth and development.

One good source of lauric acid is the cocoanut.

The best way to get it is in the form of virgin cocoanut oil.

It is not something to be consumed in large quantities, but a small daily dose is actually suggested by several of the modern nutritional and diet gurus.

This oil is used in many other countries and was once more popular here in the U.S., but became a victim of the war on saturated fats.

It was replaced with trans fats, ironically enough, which it turns out are far worse for us.

Do a Google search some time on cocoanut oil, and you will be amazed at how much comes up.

It has even been associated with claims of curing diseases.

It has been associated with helping against microbial organism infections, for one. I found this online article without looking to hard on this subject:

Fortunately ***coconut oil and other lauric oils***, as well as oregano oil, have recently been the object of study in the Georgetown University laboratory of Dr. Harry Preuss in the United States and this research has resulted in several published peer reviewed papers appearing in toxicology journals in 2005.

The antimicrobial properties of both volatile aromatic oils such as originum (oregano) oil and medium chain fatty acids such as lauric acid and its derivative monolaurin from coconut oil have shown promise in these studies. As noted by these researchers, originum oil, used as a food-flavoring agent, possesses a broad spectrum of antimicrobial activity due, at least in part, to its high content of phenolic derivatives such as carvacrol and thymol. Also, lauric acid, which is present in heavy concentrations in coconut oil, forms monolaurin in the animal body and this derivative of lauric acid can inhibit the growth of many pathogenic microorganisms.

REFERENCES

1. Preuss HG, Echard B, Enig M, Brook I, Elliott TB. Minimum inhibitory concentrations of herbal essential oils and monolaurin for gram-positive and gram-negative bacteria. *Molecular Cell Biochemistry*. 2005;272:29-34.

2. Preuss HG, Echard B, Dadgar A, Talpur N, Manohar V, Enig M, Bagchi D, Ingram C. Effects of Essential Oils and Monolaurin on *Staphylococcus aureus*: In Vitro and in Vivo Studies. *Toxicology Mechanisms and Methods* 2005;15:279-285.

About the Author

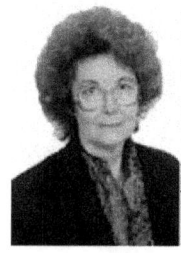

Mary G. Enig, PhD is an expert of international renown in the field of lipid biochemistry. She has headed a number of studies on the content and effects of *trans* fatty acids in America and Israel, and has successfully challenged government assertions that dietary animal fat causes cancer and heart disease.

I also found some claims that this oil could help people with thyroid issues, though any claims that it could actually "cure hypothyroidism" are certainly an exaggeration at best.

Not all nutrition "experts" are on board with the concepts mentioned, as evidenced here in an excerpt taken from Andrew Weil's website:

"Coconut oil is one of the few saturated fats that doesn't come from animals, but like other saturated fats can raise cholesterol levels and, therefore, should play only a very limited role, if any, in your diet. In the past, it was widely used in movie popcorn, candy bars and commercial baked goods but was phased out of many of them because of consumer opposition to unhealthy tropical oils.

Now coconut oil is being promoted as a weight loss aid; it is also touted in a book by a naturopathic doctor. The rationale goes something like this: as a source of medium-chain triglycerides (MCT), coconut oil isn't stored in the body as fat as readily as oils composed of long-chain triglycerides (LCT). Some research from McGill University in Canada suggests that this is true; *MCTs also boost metabolism and satiety*, and therefore may promote weight loss when they replace LCTs in the diet. Because they are so easily digested, MCTs are given in hospitals to provide nourishment for critically ill people who have trouble digesting fat.

Promoters also note that coconut oil is high in lauric acid and contains trace amounts of caprylic acid, both of which appear to have antiviral and antifungal properties, and support immune function. Lauric acid is actually present in breast milk; infants convert it to a substance called monolaurin that protects them from infections. These two fatty acids and their effects on health are being studied, but for now, we don't have any evidence suggesting that coconut oil is better for you than other saturated fats. The benefits of coconut oil in the diet, if any, are likely to be minimal, and until we have more and better evidence about coconut oil's effect of metabolism and potential role in promoting weight loss, I do not recommend using it".

Andrew Weil, M.D.

Perhaps Dr Weil is erring on the side of caution here, not wishing people to over-use this product because it is a saturated fat, after all. Make up your own mind.

Maybe you can research this some more on your own. I actually tried a teaspoon a day, taken with my vitamins in the morning, and it did seem to give an energy boost, if nothing else.

On the other hand, this well known author had this to say:

From: The Weight Loss Cure They Don't Want You To Know About by **Kevin Trudeau**.

The Weight Loss Cure Protocol: Phase I -- (1-10)

Extra Virgin Raw Coconut Oil. This is now readily available in most stores. Use this as your fat of choice in cooking. Take two teaspoons per day. This is *proven to stimulate metabolism, improve digestion, and help release fat cells. It also gently stimulates the thyroid."*

Keep in mind that in the book mentioned above, Kevin lists this among a number of other things that should be used together for best results.

As with any supplement, we must be cautious when the people touting the benefits just happen to have a financial interest in it. University studies and studies by medical institutions and the like tend to be more objective and reliable in that regard.

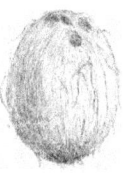

Over the counter appetite suppressants

This is an area that does not seem to be talked about much by a lot of the diet & nutrition experts. Yet, it is a multi-billion dollar industry, and something that many people trying to lose pounds resort to commonly. I feel that most of these are potentially more harmful than they are beneficial, and I think most of the experts are on the same page, thus their lack of discussing this area very much. Caffeine is found in many, along with various other stimulants. Caffeine itself is not too bad, and some studies have even suggested it to be good for us, in moderation. It does have appetite suppressant and mild thermogenic qualities. Two or three cups of coffee daily will probably not hurt you, unless you have high blood pressure, heart palpitations or sensitivity to the effects of caffeine beyond the norm.

The problem with many of the OTC products is the *lack of regulation* of these products. A list of these products that contain large doses of pharmaceutical stimulants, diuretics, etc, has recently been circulated in the media, and the list is quite long. A lot of these items make claims to contain all natural ingredients, yet this is far from the truth. You are much better off with the herbal products listed previously.

In fact, the FDA recently posted this warning on their website about tainted OTC weight loss products:

FDA Uncovers Additional Tainted Weight Loss Products
Agency alerts consumers to the finding of new undeclared drug ingredients

The U.S. Food and Drug Administration is expanding, for the second time, its nationwide alert to consumers about tainted weight loss products containing undeclared, active pharmaceutical ingredients.

The FDA has identified additional weight loss products (Herbal Xenicol, Slimbionic, and Xsvelten) and new undeclared active pharmaceutical ingredients (fenproporex, fluoxetine, furosemide, and cetilistat). The current list now includes the following 72 products:

2 Day Diet	Fatloss Slimming	Slim 3 in 1 M18 Royal Diet
2 Day Diet Slim Advance	GMP	Slim 3 in 1 Slim Formula
2x Powerful Slimming	Herbal Xenicol	Slim Burn
3 Day Diet	Imelda Fat Reducer	Slim Express 4 in 1
3 Days Fit	Imelda Perfect Slim	Slim Express 360
3x Slimming Power	JM Fat Reducer	Slim Fast*
5x Imelda Perfect Slimming	Lida DaiDaihua	Slim Tech
7 Day Herbal Slim	Meili	Slim Up
7 Days Diet	Meizitang	Slim Waist Formula
7 Diet	Miaozi MeiMaoQianZiJiaoNang	Slim Waistline
7 Diet Day/Night Formula	Miaozi Slim Capsules	Slimbionic
8 Factor Diet	Natural Model	Sliminate
Eight Factor Diet	Perfect Slim	Slimming Formula
21 Double Slim	Perfect Slim 5x	Somotrim
24 Hours Diet	Perfect Slim Up	Starcaps
999 Fitness Essence	Phyto Shape	Super Fat Burner
BioEmagrecim	Powerful Slim	Superslim
Body Creator	ProSlim Plus	Super Slimming
Body Shaping	Reduce Weihgt	Trim 2 Plus
Body Slimming	Royal Slimming Formula	Triple Slim
Cosmo Slim	Sana Plus	Venom Hyperdrive 3.0
Extrim Plus	Slim 3 in 1	Waist Strength Formula
Extrim Plus 24 Hour Reburn	Slim 3 in 1 Extra Slim Formula	Xsvelten

Fasting Diet	Slim 3 in 1 Extra Slim Waist Formula	Zhen de Shou

* This product should not be confused with the line of meal replacement and related products that are marketed as conventional foods under the brand name "Slim-Fast®". The manufacturer of Slim-Fast®, Unilever United States, Inc., maintains that the Slim Fast product which appears on this list is not in any way associated with, sponsored or approved by, or otherwise related in any way to the Slim-Fast® brand of meal replacement and related products.

"These tainted weight loss products pose a great risk to public health because they contain undeclared ingredients and, in some cases, contain prescription drugs in amounts that greatly exceed maximum recommended dosages," said Janet Woodcock, M.D., director of the FDA's Center for Drug Evaluation and Research. "Consumers have no way of knowing that these products contain dangerous drugs that could cause serious consequences to their health."

On Dec. 22, 2008, the FDA warned consumers not to purchase or consume 28 different products marketed for weight loss. On Jan. 8, 2009, the FDA expanded the list of tainted weight loss products to include 41 additional tainted products. The FDA will continue to update this list as warranted.

The products listed above, some of which are marketed as dietary supplements, are promoted and sold on various Web sites and in some retail stores and beauty salons. Some of the products claim to be "natural" or to contain only "herbal" ingredients, but actually contain potentially harmful ingredients not listed on the products' labels or in promotional advertisements. These products have not been approved by the FDA, are illegal, and include the following undeclared active pharmaceutical ingredients:

- sibutramine (an appetite suppressant available by prescription only and a controlled substance)
- fenproporex – a controlled substance not approved for marketing in the United States;
- fluoxetine – an antidepressant available by prescription only;
- bumetanide – a potent diuretic available by prescription only;
- furosemide – a potent diuretic available by prescription only;

- rimonabant – a drug not approved for marketing in the United States;
- cetilistat – an experimental obesity drug not approved for marketing in the United States;
- phenytoin – an anti-seizure medication available by prescription only; and
- phenolphthalein – a solution used in chemical experiments and a suspected cancer-causing agent that is not approved for marketing in the United States.

The FDA has inspected a number of companies associated with the sale of these illegal products and is currently seeking product recalls. Based on the FDA's inspections and the companies' inadequate responses to recall requests, the FDA may take additional enforcement steps, such as issuing warning letters or initiating seizures, injunctions, or criminal charges.

The FDA advises consumers who have used any products containing these ingredients to stop taking them and consult their health care professional immediately. The FDA also encourages consumers to seek guidance from a health care professional before purchasing weight loss products.

The health risks posed by these products can be very serious and include high blood pressure, seizures, tachycardia (rapid heartbeat), palpitations, heart attack, and stroke. Sibutramine, a controlled substance, was found in many of these products at levels much higher than the maximum daily dosage for Meridia, the only FDA-approved drug product containing sibutramine. These higher levels of sibutramine can increase the incidence and severity of these health risks. Fenproporex, another controlled substance, can cause arrhythmia and possible sudden death.

Health care professionals and consumers should report serious adverse events (side effects) or product quality problems to the FDA's MedWatch Adverse Event Reporting program either online, by regular mail, fax or phone.

- Online
- Regular Mail: use postage-paid FDA form 3500 and mail to MedWatch, 5600 Fishers Lane, Rockville, MD 20852-9787
- Fax: 800-FDA-0178
- Phone: 800-FDA-1088

For more information:

Information on FDA's Initiative Against Contaminated Weight Loss Products

To learn more about the FDA's initiative against unapproved drugs see the FDA's Compliance Policy Guide at: http://www.fda.gov/cder/Guidance/6911fnl.htm.

For drug safety information, see: FDA's Drug Safety Initiative.

-

Cleansing protocols

Cleansing in this context is talking about detoxifying or cleaning out the intestines, bowels and other parts of the digestive tract. There are a number of commercial formulae in addition to the older herbal remedies for this. Claims are made for great weight loss using these methods, which are typically greatly exaggerated. Weight loss does occur, largely in the form of loss of fluids. This weight loss is also typically only temporary, unfortunately. On the brighter side, intestinal/digestive cleansing methods can remove harmful bacteria, toxic substances like partially un-digested food that has fermented, and other such nastiness.

In that regard, it may be worthwhile to try a cleansing protocol at the start of a new eating/diet program, just to provide a "clean palette" Just keep in mind that that initial quick weight loss will probably be short-lived, and don't get stressed about it too much.

You may want to try the more pleasant forms of ridding the body of excess fluids, such as the sauna or a steam bath. You actually burn off some calories in addition to sweating out the fluids when you sit in a sauna, so it is beneficial in more ways than one.

Of course, you must limit your time in the sauna or steam bath, as spending too long a time in either can cause problems, especially for those with heart conditions or other health concerns. At the very least, these can be a great way to relax after a traditional workout if you are in good health. Also consider that the heart rate goes up while using the sauna, which burns calories as we mentioned.

Steam makes you sweat like a sauna does, but is a moist heat instead of a dry heat. Like the sauna, it is said to relax the muscles and it is also claimed to be good for the skin. Home steam showers have become popular in the high-end bathrooms of modern homes. There is a potential negative to these, according to some health authors.

Typical household water from the tap contains high levels of chlorine, unless the water is properly filtered or treated. Chlorine is not good to ingest either through drinking it or by absorbing it through the pores of the skin. When chlorine is "atomized" by being converted to steam, it becomes easier for it to get into your system when you take a steam bath or steam shower. This may nullify any potential benefits gained.

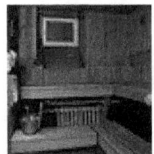

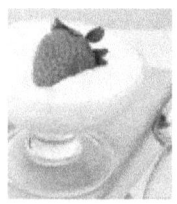

Chapter Six

Healthy Bacteria

We have mentioned the subject of intestinal bacteria; we should mention that they are not all bad. You may have noticed the recent trend with all the yogurt companies touting the beneficial bacteria in their products, and how they help to promote a healthy and balanced "flora" in the gut.

Probiotics is a rather hot term that has been getting thrown around a lot lately. Probiotics are beneficial micro-organisms that help in the proper absorption and digestion of our food. They keep food from rotting or fermenting in the gut.

Here is an excerpt from "medicinenet.com" website on the subject:

"Good" Bacteria Foods: Health or Hype?

Probiotics may be a healthy addition to your diet
By Kathleen Zelman, MPH, RD, LD
WebMD Weight Loss Clinic - Expert Column

March 10, 2006 -- There has been a significant buzz on television commercials and in the media making a strong case that everyone needs to add probiotics into their diets for good health. Faith Popcorn, trend predictor, noted probiotics as one of the hottest food trends for 2006. Are you confused by terms like probiotics that sound more like a chemistry experiment than a dietary supplement? You're not alone.
Probiotics are the latest in the category of good-for-you foods. Basically, they are "good" bacteria added to foods or occurring naturally in certain yogurts, fermented dairy drinks, and in supplement form. Probiotics have been used as a form of treatment for a variety of gastrointestinal diseases

including irritable bowel, lactose intolerance, traveler's diarrhea, and antibiotic-induced diarrhea.

How do they work? Scientists are not exactly sure but surmise that the good bacteria replace or crowd out the germs or bad bacteria in the intestinal tract. Another theory is that the good bugs keep the intestinal tract acidic to the point where bad bugs can't survive. Our digestive tracts are lined with more than 400 different kinds of good bacteria that help fight off infection and keep us healthy. The largest group of good bacteria is the one found in yogurt. By consuming foods with probiotics, you can increase the number of healthy bacteria, boost your immunity, and promote a healthy digestive system.

I eat organic yogurt on a regular, if not daily basis. The benefits to the organic stuff are higher protein content and lack of ugly additives such as high fructose corn syrup. While you may consider adding any old yogurt to your diet as being a step towards better health, not all yogurts are created equal. Also, note that the newer "Gogurt" and things like that may reel in the kids attention, and get them to eat it, this is inferior to the real thing, in terms of having less protein (typically only a couple of grams per serving), and more artificial sweeteners and additives.

Kefir is another food/beverage that contains healthy bacteria. There is actually a website I found describing the differences, and these folks are apparently huge fans of Kefir.

Their home page reads as follows:

Both kefir and yogurt are cultured milk products...
...but they contain different types of beneficial bacteria. Yogurt contains transient beneficial bacteria that keep the digestive system clean and provide food for the friendly bacteria that reside there. But kefir can actually colonize the intestinal tract, a feat that yogurt cannot match.

Kefir contains several major strains of friendly bacteria not commonly found in yogurt, Lactobacillus Caucasus, Leuconostoc, Acetobacter species, and Streptococcus species.

It also contains beneficial yeasts, such as Saccharomyces kefir and Torula kefir, which dominate, control and eliminate destructive pathogenic yeasts in the body. They do so by penetrating the mucosal lining where unhealthy yeast and bacteria reside, forming a virtual SWAT team that housecleans and strengthens the intestines. Hence, the body becomes more efficient in resisting such pathogens as E. coli and intestinal parasites.

Kefir's active yeast and bacteria provide more nutritive value than yogurt by helping digest the foods that you eat and by keeping the colon environment clean and healthy.

Because the curd size of kefir is smaller than yogurt, it is also easier to digest, which makes it a particularly excellent, nutritious food for babies, invalids and the elderly, as well as a remedy for digestive disorders.

Read more here:

http://www.kefir.net/kefiryogurt.htm

You can purchase this amazing stuff at regular grocers, health food stores, or you can actually make your own!

Chapter Seven

Is Cheating O.K.?

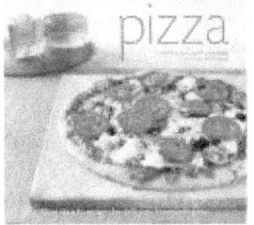

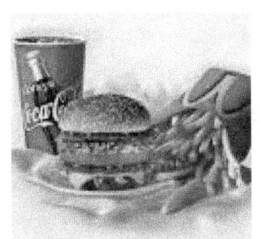

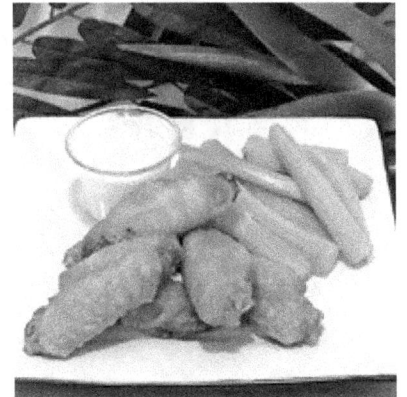

Firstly, what do I mean by cheating? Well, in this case I'm talking about cheating on your diet. Maybe it's a bowl of good old fashioned, full strength, full fat ice cream, or several slices of pizza with all the fatty, but delicious toppings you love. It could even be a full day of eating whatever you enjoy (within reason, of course).There are quite a few experts saying that this may not only be less harmful than most have thought, but it may even be very healthy and helpful. It can help on a couple of different levels; one psychological and the other physical.

On the mental level, it can help one stay on track throughout the week, if a reward during the weekend can be looked forward to. This holds true in many areas of life, and it holds true for maintaining a healthy nutritional lifestyle as well. Having some deliciously decadent food in moderation, on occasion should not be associated with feelings of guilt or failure, even for those that really need to lose weight.

Perhaps an even more compelling reason has to do with a hormone called *Leptin.*

The following is a university description of this hormone and its effects:

From:

http://www.vivo.colostate.edu/hbooks/pathphys/endocrine/bodyweight/leptin.html

Leptin

Leptin (from the Greek *leptos*, meaning thin) is a protein hormone with important effects in regulating body weight, metabolism and reproductive function. Leptin is expressed predominantly by adipocytes, which fits with the idea that body weight is sensed as the total mass of fat in the body. Smaller amounts of leptin are also secreted by cells in the epithelium of the stomach and in the placenta. Leptin receptors are highly expressed in areas of the hypothalamus known to be important in regulating body weight, as well as in T lymphocytes and vascular endothelial cells.

Physiologic Effects of leptin

Regulation of Food Intake, Energy Expenditure and Body Weight

Leptin is an important component in the long term regulation of body weight. Recent studies with obese and non-obese humans demonstrated a strong positive correlation of serum leptin concentrations with percentage of body fat, and also that there was a higher concentration of ob mRNA in fat from obese compared to thin subjects. It appears that as adipocytes increase in size due to accumulation of triglyceride, they synthesize more and more leptin. *In essence, leptin provides the body with an index of nutritional status.*

Leptin's effects on body weight are mediated through effects on hypothalamic centers that control feeding behavior and hunger, body temperature and energy expenditure.. As depicted in the graph below, weight loss resulting from administration of leptin appears to result from a combination of at least two fundamental effects:

- **Decreased hunger and food consumption** mediated at least in part by inhibition of neuropeptide Y synthesis. Neuropeptide Y is a very potent stimulator of feeding behavior.

- **Increased energy expenditure**, measured as increased oxygen consumption, higher body temperature and loss of adipose tissue mass.

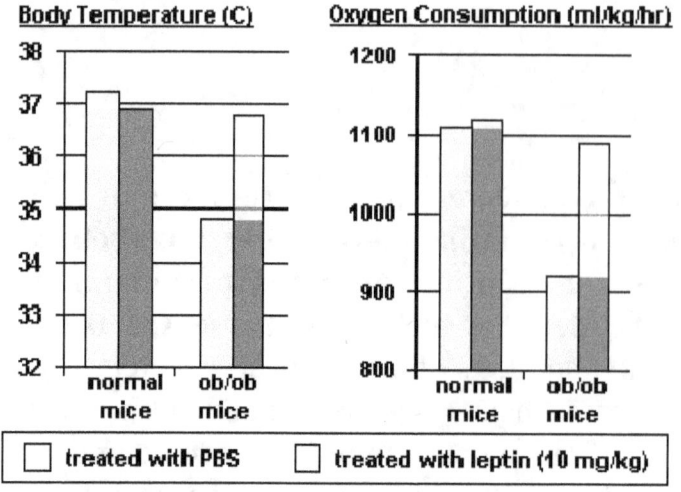

(Adapted from Pellymounter et al., Science 269:540, 1995)

As expected, injections of leptin into db/db mice, which lack the leptin receptor, had no effect. When leptin was given to normal mice, they lost weight, showed ***profound depletion of adipose tissue and manifest increases in lean mass.***

The mechanisms by which leptin exerts its effects on metabolism are largely unknown and are likely quite complex. In contrast to dieting, which results in loss of both fat and lean mass, treatment with leptin promotes lipolysis in adipose tissue, but has no apparent effect on lean tissue.

.

Control of Leptin Synthesis and Secretion

The amount of leptin expressed by adipocytes correlates well with the lipid content of the cells. Once synthesized, leptin is secreted through a constitutive pathway and not stored in the cell.

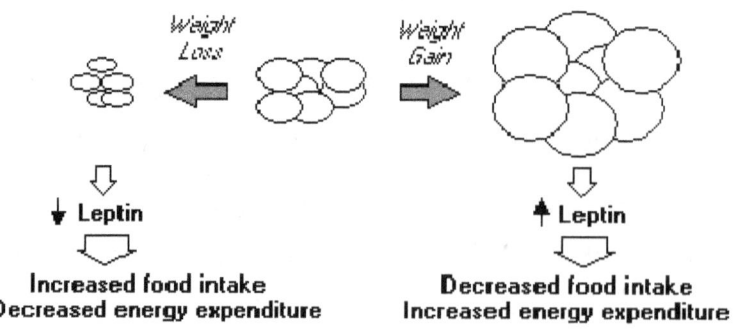

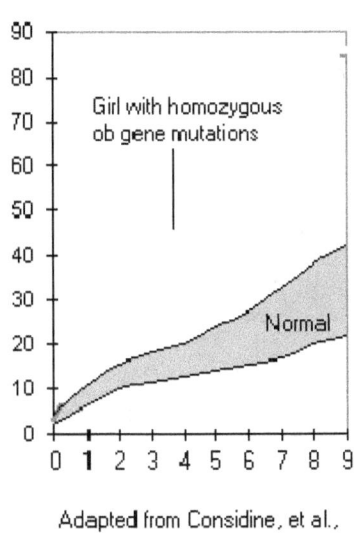

Girl with homozygous ob gene mutations

Normal

Adapted from Considine, et al., New Eng J Med 334:292, 1996.

At this time, the mechanisms responsible for regulating leptin expression in adipocytes are unknown. It is likely that a number of hormones modulate ob gene expression, including glucocorticoids and insulin.

Disease States

Mice with inactivating mutations in the gene encoding leptin or its receptor have indistinguishable, recessive phenotypes of obesity, with roughly three times the body weight and five times the fat mass of normal mice. They also manifest diabetes, and show cold intolerance, depressed immune function and infertility.

Blood concentrations of Leptin are usually increased in obese humans, suggesting that they are in some way insensitive to leptin, rather than suffering from leptin deficiency. Mutations in ob or db genes appear to be a very rare cause of morbid obesity in humans, but both have been described. The effect of such mutations on body weight is dramatic, as shown here. The figure to the right depicts the growth curve for a young girl found to have homozygous inactivating mutations of the ob gene, contrasted to normal children (2nd to 98th percentiles).

Leptin therapy will require either frequent injections or genetic therapy, precluding its use for trivial purposes.

References and Reviews

- Cherhab FF, Mounzih K, Lu R, Lim ME: Early onset of reproductive function in normal female mice treated with leptin. Science 275:88, 1997.
- Clement K, Vaisse C, Lahlou N, et al: A mutation in the human leptin receptor gene causes obesity and pituitary dysfunction. Nature 392:398, 1998.
- Considine RV, Sinha MK, Heiman ML etc: Serum immunoreactive-leptin concentrations in normal-weight and obese humans. New Eng J Med 334:292, 1996.
- Friedman JM, Halaas JL: Leptin and the regulation of body weight in mammals. Nature 395:763, 1998.
- Halaas JL, Gajiwala KS, Maffel M, etc: Weight-reducing effects of the plasma protein encoded by the obese gene. Science 269:543, 1995.
- Montague CT, Faroozi IS, Whitehead JP, etc: Congenital leptin deficiency is associated with severe early-onset obesity in humans. Nature 387:903, 1997.
- Pelleymounter MA, Cullen MJ, Baker MB, etc: Effects of the *obese* gene product on body weight regulation in ob/ob mice. Science 269:540, 1995.
- Zhang Y, Proenca R, Maffei M, etc: Positional cloning of the mouse obese gene and its human homologue. Nature 372:425, 1994.

So what does all of this scientific jargon mean for the lay person? The most meaningful thing to learn from the above information is that leptin is a very important hormone for those trying to shed fat. While getting leptin injections is not a real option for most of us, is there a way to naturally stimulate or regulate this hormone to attain its benefits?

There have been studies suggesting that a calorie restricted diet leads ultimately to reduced Leptin secretion by the body. It has also been suggested that this is largely what causes weight loss to suddenly or at least gradually come to a halt after initial losses.

The bad news

The feedback mechanism of the body's hormonal system detects that calories have been restricted and it responds by cutting down on Leptin production/secretion. This happens over a period of time.

The good news

The good news is that this response is not only reversible, but the reversal comes about relatively quickly in relation to the time period it takes for the initial response to happen. What that means is that "falling off the wagon" on a regular, perhaps weekly basis, may be beneficial to Leptin regulation. In other words, your body will respond to a high calorie, high fat meal fairly quickly by producing and/or secreting more Leptin, which will now stay elevated for a while and allow your re-restricted diet to start working as desired again, and you will lose more fat again. This is an example of how modern scientific findings have shown us that the old concepts that losing weight is simply about reducing calories and/or burning more calories is a huge over-simplification of the many processes involved.

Chapter Eight

Growing your own organic garden

What a tremendous way to "kill two birds with one stone"!
Gardening is a great form of exercise, for starters.
You will get more fresh air, and the food you grow will arrive at the table as fresh as can be, delicious and full of nutrients.
If you can avoid chemicals in the growing process, such as insecticides, you will have raised truly organic food, also.
It can be a little intimidating starting out in this field (no pun intended), but it does not have to be very complicated, really.
Choose easy to grow items at first, like tomatoes, peppers and zucchini.
A small plot of ground, a couple of simple hand tools and some packs of seeds or already started young plants will get you on your way. There is plenty of information available online, on T.V., and in books and periodicals that can tell you everything you need to know about this subject.
I grew some tomatoes last year, and this year I have planted lettuce, onions, carrots, peppers, eggplant, peas and zucchini.
It is very satisfying to pick fresh veggies from your own plot for your dinner table, so give it some serious thought.

 If growing your own produce seems a bit too labor intensive, and/or you just don't feel that you have a green thumb, you can always opt to purchase produce from a local farmer's market if you are blessed enough to have one nearby.
Another option that is becoming available lately is farm co-ops.
Local growers will provide in-season produce to people that pre-buy "shares" in their agri-business. This is a win-win for the business and the purchaser.

The only real down side to this is that you can only get "in-season"
items that come into season according to your local weather, etc.
This really is a more natural way of eating and was the traditional way in the
"good old days".
Lately, we get produce grown all over the world and shipped to us so that we
can have pretty much anything our little hearts desire at any time of year.
This too has its downsides.
Produce that is grown in other countries and shipped to our markets is
chemically altered to maintain freshness, and is not nearly as good as that
picked fresh from your local farm.
You must also keep in mind that even your local farm may use other than
true organic methods. Pesticides and other chemicals may be used,
especially on the larger farms.

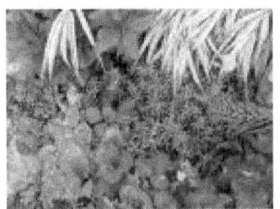

Chapter Nine

Foraging

Foraging for wild food is another great idea; but be sure to learn to properly identify your quarry if you decide to try this.

There are field guides, and some experts offer field trips to educate the newbie in this area.

There are many fairly easy to identify wild foods that can probably be harvested right in your backyard.

Cattails have edible shoots in the spring and edible pollen as well.

Day lilies have edible parts, as do the common dandelion and some other plants considered as weeds.

You will also be getting in some exercise walking through the woods, picking berries, etc.

In the fall, mast crops such as chestnuts, walnuts and other nuts will be available and provide a great source of protein at no cost.

Mushrooms grow in the wild and certain varieties are foraged for by experts and are quite expensive to purchase.

One of the problems with harvesting wild mushrooms is that there are lots of look-alikes to the edible and delicious varieties that are actually deadly.

I would not eat any wild mushrooms without an absolutely positive I.D.! It would probably be very beneficial for the newcomer to foraging to become very educated on the subject, and perhaps get some hands-on training from true experts in the field.

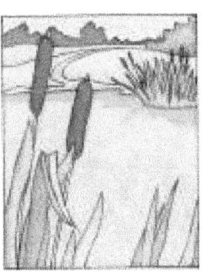

Cattails have edible parts

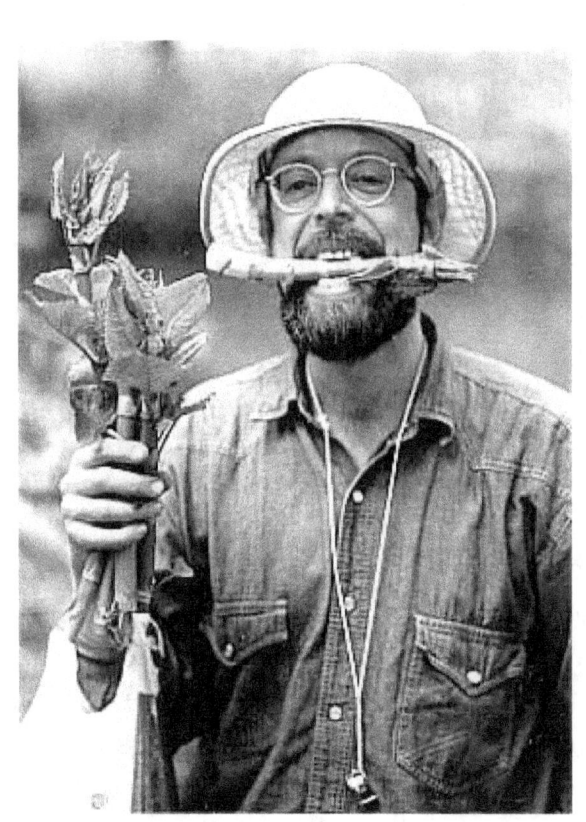

Chapter Ten

Getting started with exercise and activities

I think that a big part of the problem for most overweight folks
Is that they find conventional exercise modes boring, tedious, or downright torture. People join gyms, pay up front for a year or more of membership and then quit after a short time. Most large commercial gym owners love this, as they get money for nothing, and never run out of room at the facility. Getting and staying fit is a life long thing, not something you do for a few months to "get back in shape" and then go back to the old routine that got you out of shape in the first place. Get off the roller coaster!

If you have been relatively sedentary for a long time, just joining a gym for 2 years and expecting yourself to go and train as needed for that entire time is not doable for most folks. It requires a whole lot of will power, which if you had in the first place would have kept you out of trouble.

You have to start out easy, make reasonable short term goals that are very attainable *for you* and gradually build from there.

There are bound to be a few activities on the list of 50 above that you actually enjoy and find relaxing or recreational and fun.

Maybe there are some things you have never even tried, but that sound at least remotely appealing. Give some new things a whirl, you may be pleasantly surprised.

Taking walks in the outdoors with your spouse or a friend, even your pooch, can be a very enjoyable way to get your exercise in.

Many fitness programs are built almost entirely around walking.

Walking is free, requires little in the way of equipment, and virtually anyone can do it.

Even if you start out simply walking around the block, it's a step in the right direction. You can begin with a walk around the block 2 or 3 days per week, and then add days and/or distance over time until the calories burned and the benefits gained really start to snowball.

On the other hand, if you go out on your first workout and walk or jog several miles by forcing yourself to do it, you will not enjoy it very much, you will get sore afterwards and probably stay sore for days, and you will become discouraged about the entire idea.

Then you are back to square one. Be patient and enjoy the ride.

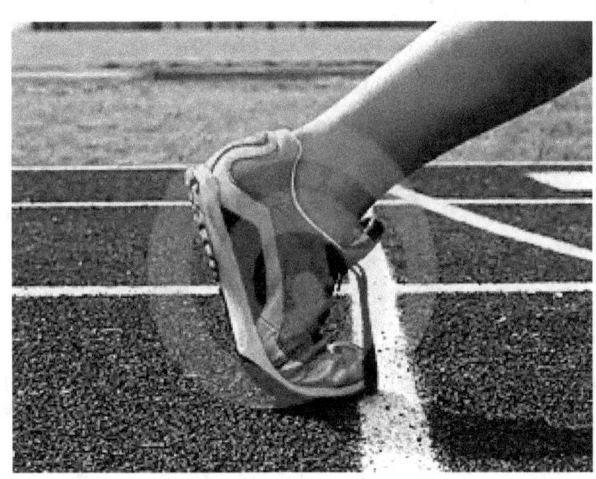

Adding steps

One of the listed items under "50 ways with exercise", number 2 in fact, was adding steps. What exactly did I mean by that?

Pedometers are nifty little tools that are an inexpensive way of tracking every step you take during your typical day.

Just being aware of how many steps you take will help you to make some healthy adjustments.

The better quality pedometers will even report calories burned and miles or kilometers logged, based on some setup information from the user.

When you become more aware of your daily steps, you may start trying to increase your steps gradually, by parking a bit farther away from the store you are going into, your workplace, etc. for one. Taking the steps instead of the elevator or escalator (see item one on our list), not only adds steps but is even better than walking on flat surfaces, and gets the heart rate up a little more. Taking a walk during breaks, at lunch, etc., will add still more steps to the daily total. These things do not require a huge time expenditure yet can go a long way towards your calorie burning goals.

You typically have to "calibrate" a pedometer to make sure it reports correctly for your stride length, weight, and so forth.

This is not too difficult. You can go even more "high tech"
with a heart rate monitor watch and its accompanying strap that picks up the signal from your heart and transmits it to the watch.

These are more expensive than a simple pedometer, but also are far more useful and versatile.

The most expensive versions of these report actual heart rate, can tell you if you are staying within a specific zone, give calories burned, mileage and even contain an onboard GPS device!

You can wear it during any activity (except swimming, duh) and get the calories burned report after you are done.

You can set up workout profiles, heart rate zones, etc, and have the watch alarm activate when you are not in the zone or something is not going according to the plan.

Anything that makes tracking progress and even makes it more fun is a welcome addition to the trainee.

These devices even serve as a safety measure, telling you if your heart rate has gone over the suggested maximum.

You might think this would be obvious to the exerciser, but this is not always the case.

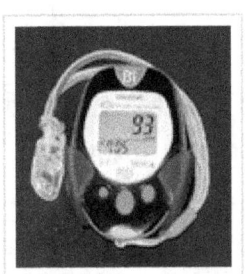

Playing Games

Until recently, nobody would claim that playing a video game was actually a form of exercise. That has changed now.

The Wii fit games have introduced a whole new world of possibilities.

Is playing video fitness games likely to replace normal gym visits and conventional workouts? This is probably not likely, any time soon, anyway. But for the sedentary, these games are a great way to start doing something physical without getting crazy.

To be sure, bodybuilders and hardcore fitness buffs will not be challenged much by the games, but they might make a fun addition to the workout schedule. Manufacturers of real gym equipment like treadmills and stationary bikes are also cashing in on this trend, and putting interactive video screens on their equipment which make workouts more fun.

You might be trying to flee from a dragon trying to scorch you, or be in pursuit of a bad guy ahead of you as you run or ride the bike.

This is a pretty cool concept, I think, and one that is bound to catch on in our modern society.

Other game makers are bound to jump on the bandwagon anytime now also, considering the popularity of the Wii.

My wife and I are getting a system this week, as a matter of fact, and I'm looking forward to some fun workouts at home with the misses.

Rowing, Sculling, and Kayaking

All of the above from our list are similar and potentially fun to do, while at the same time getting some fresh air and sunshine while you exercise. Using a rowing machine certainly works, but in my opinion not nearly as fun as the real thing, like most things in life.

If you happen to be a fisherman, like me, you can use a canoe, small rowboat or kayak to paddle yourself into some great fish holding water and get a workout on the way. With a bit of good fortune, you'll get another workout reeling in some big fish!

Who could ask for more?

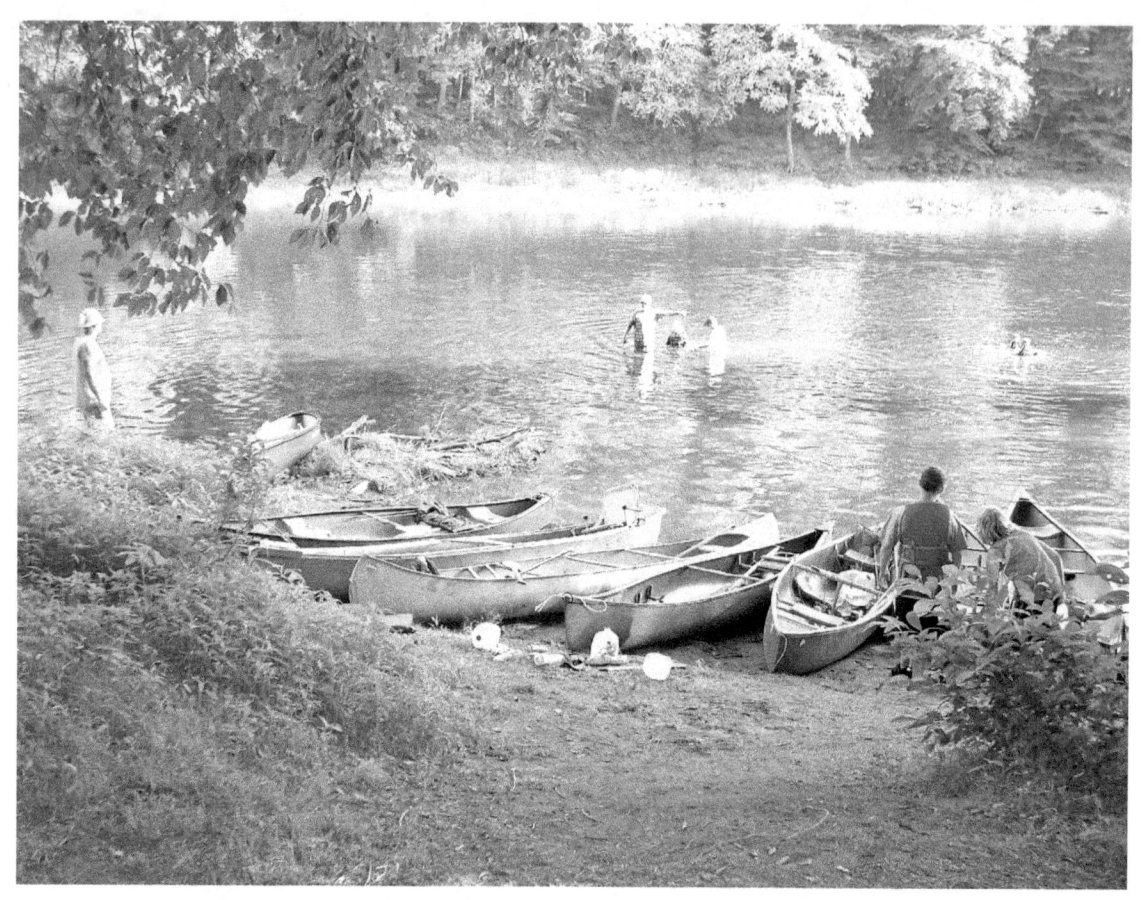

Dancing

While I must admit this is not my forte', many folks find this a very pleasurable form of exercise, and again this is not something that is expensive to get involved in.

Dancing can burn lots of calories and be very beneficial to the cardio-respiratory system.

Line dancing; belly dancing, ballroom dancing, free style dancing like Elaine on the Seinfeld show… its all good!

There are some types of dancing, like the Russian Cossack's dance, that are tremendously challenging and good forms of exercise. Essentially, you remain in a full squat position with arms crossed, and then kick each leg out in an alternating fashion.

This may not be popular on the modern dance floor, and you are not likely to see it done by celebrities on "Dancing with the Stars",

But it may well be the best exercise form of dance you could ever find.

Some of the old school strongmen even practiced this in their training routines.

See my earlier book "Forgotten Secrets of the Old Time Strongmen"

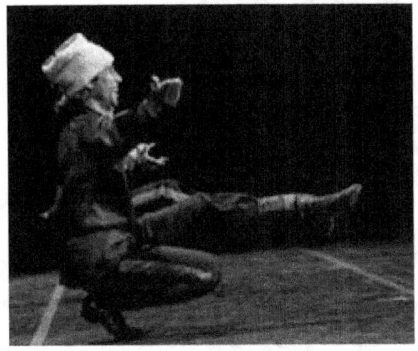

A word about Interval Training

I mentioned interval training with walking and jogging or running in our list above, but there are numerous types of interval training.

Weight training can be done using this concept, and so can bodyweight training. It really just boils down to varying the pace of the exercise from relatively easy to very challenging, and then back to easy. This type of training can be very useful for those trying to shed some fat, as there is a pretty high "burn rate" associated with it.

Another advantage to this mode of training is that you get a continued burn for a considerable time after the workout.

This has been tagged with the acronym EPOC, which stands for excess post exercise oxygen consumption.

Some trainers have come up with other catch words for this, like "Turbulence Training", for one.

There is a misconception that low intensity, long duration style cardio workouts are superior for fat loss to higher intensity workouts of shorter duration.

If you have been on one of the more sophisticated treadmills at a commercial gym, there is typically a display that shows a certain intensity level (correlates with your heart rate) as being in the optimal "fat-burning zone". It may also tell you that you must stay in that zone for 30-40 minutes or more to burn a significant number of calories.

While this is essentially the truth, it can be a bit misleading, really.

The thing is, once you step off the treadmill after this slower paced workout, the calorie burning stops pretty much immediately.

On the other hand, if you really push hard and work up a sweat by running up simulated hills and or by running faster, you will continue to burn calories well after you step off the treadmill.

You may not see the calories burned on the treadmill display, and in fact it will probably tell you that you have burned less calories if your workout was relatively short, but in the long run, you will have burned more with the combination of calories burned both during and then ***after*** the initial workout.

Interval training provides the best of both worlds, because you can train longer by taking slower paced breathers, and get in the high intensity stuff in spurts. You burn more calories during and after the workout this way, and you still don't get completely "wasted" from all out exertion for the time period.

To apply this method to weight training, many trainers suggest doing exercises for a set time period and perhaps an equal period of rest, rather than doing a certain number of repetitions.

Calisthenics or bodyweight only exercises also lend themselves well to this concept.

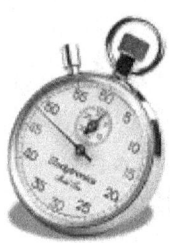

Some examples of Interval Training

One of the simpler forms of this is used in a program called "couch to 5k", which takes the trainee from being largely sedentary to the point where he or she can actually be expected to compete in a 5k race. The idea is to start out with just walking, and then you start adding in short jogs during the walks. You continue to lengthen the jogging time while decreasing the walking time until you are jogging/running the full distance required.

Of course, you can just continue to keep switching back and forth between walking and jogging and make your workouts longer and longer, as a good variation of this method.

The beauty of it is that you can do it completely at your own pace and build up as gradually as you feel comfortable with.

To apply it to a weight training workout, you could (after a light cardio warm up) pick up a pair of dumbbells as you bend into a squatting position, holding them with palms forward, and then rise up to an upright position while simultaneously thrusting the bells overhead until both arms are locked out.

You want to perform this in an explosive, fast and forceful motion, and then continue repetitions for about 30 seconds (stopwatch or watch/clock with second hands needed here). You would then stop and rest for 30 seconds and follow with another "set".

You should perform at least 2 or more cycles of the exercise/rest routine or continue until you are no longer capable of doing so.

The exercise described is called the squat-press, which is really a combination of a lower body exercise with an upper body exercise.

You would ideally do another exercise that hits all the major sections of the body, such as a "lunging punch" with dumbbells.

In this movement, you would lunge forward on one leg while "punching" the bells forward at the same time. Bring the bells back to the sides as you return to the full upright position with both legs locked, and then lunge with the opposite leg as you again punch forward with the bells. Once again, continue the movement for 30 seconds and follow with an equally timed rest period, for several cycles if possible.

Several cycles each of both of these exercises would provide a quick, intense workout that hits most of the major muscle groups while burning calories during and after the workout.

Add these short workouts following a normal walk, bike ride, swim or rowing session (or whatever) and you have created a dynamo of a workout routine that does not require much of your time.

You can add exercises, sets, time or weight as you progress in strength and ability.

Calisthenics work well also, if you don't have weights or prefer an alternative to them.

Do 30 seconds of jumping jacks followed by 30 seconds of rest.

Next do 30 seconds of mountain climbers for 30 seconds with an equal rest period after.

You could add pushups along with the jumping jacks for one combined movement, or add as a separate cycle.

Running in place, jumping rope, doing chin ups, etc could all be thrown in the mix with this type of training according to your abilities and likes.

You could also mix protocols like one cycle with weights, followed by another with calisthenics or bodyweight moves.

Another option is to hit the local public jogging track that also has a jungle gym or monkey bars, etc.

You could walk or jog a lap, and then do some chin ups on the bars, or dips on the parallel bars, or whatever else is available. Mix it up and have some fun.

Isometrics, Virtual resistance training and Iso-flexing

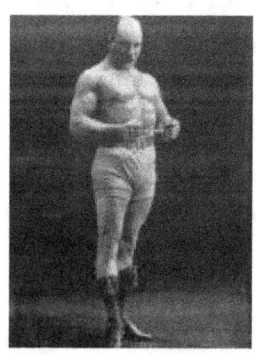

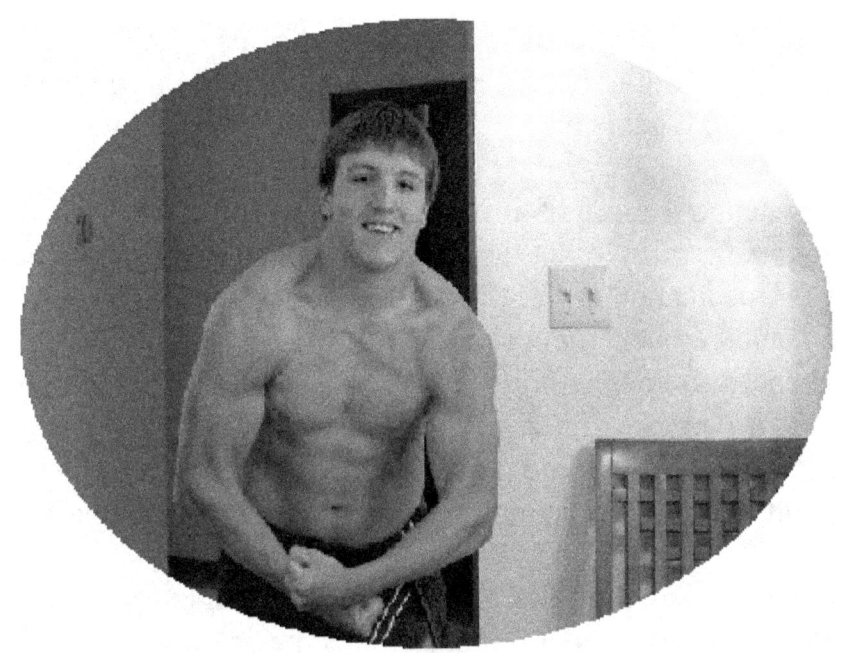

My stepson Kevin flexing

Here are a few items from the list that may not be obvious to some of you.
Isometrics is probably more familiar than the other two.
Basically, Isometrics is strength training by pushing or pulling against an immovable object, such as a wall.
One of the big benefits to isometrics is that it can be done virtually anywhere with no or very little equipment.
In fact, this author recently published a manual entitled "Autometrics, A complete manual on how to workout in your car"
I also tell about a man named Sanford Bennett in my latest book,
"The secrets of Age Defying Strength" (and how to obtain it)
Bennett penned a book on *exercising in bed* based on isometrics and flexing/relaxing the muscles.
Isometrics by itself will not burn a great deal of calories, but it does strengthen and build muscle. Since muscle tissue burns more calories than fat does, you increase your BMR by adding muscle which will enable you to burn more calories in the long run.
You can build shoulders and arms by pushing outward or upward in a doorway, or your chest, triceps and shoulders by pushing forward against the door frame.

You should do isometric movements from various points involved in the typical range of motion, because isometrics tends to build strength primarily in the position that gets held.

Virtual resistance is more of an "internal" resistance that is self generated. The **antagonistic** muscles are used to provide resistance to the working muscle(s). This is another very versatile form of training that requires no equipment and can be done just about anywhere.
Another benefit to this method is that you can "invent" imaginary exercise machines to *hit any muscle from any angle you choose.*
It sounds a little quirky to the uninitiated, I'll admit, but there are many folks who use and swear by these methods, and some use them exclusively.

Lay on a flat surface, the floor or a bench, and imagine pushing a heavy weight off your chest as in a standard bench press movement.
In fact, don't just imagine, but physically perform the exercise movement with the working muscles (chest, front deltoids or shoulders, and triceps or back of arms). Use the antagonistic muscles (back, biceps) to provide resistance to the working muscles. You can make the resistance as light or as heavy as you like, but use moderation as you get the feel of this.
You can perform any exercise you like using the method described.

Iso-flexing is simply isolating a particular muscle or muscle group and flexing it hard, as in a bodybuilder posing routine.
Hold the flexed position for 5-10 seconds or more, and try to increase the force as you continue holding the flexed position.
Once again, this can be done anywhere, and I talked about this and virtual resistance movements in the *Autometrics* manual mentioned above.
Iso-flexing can also be combined with virtual resistance and/or isometric training to create some very interesting and challenging routines.

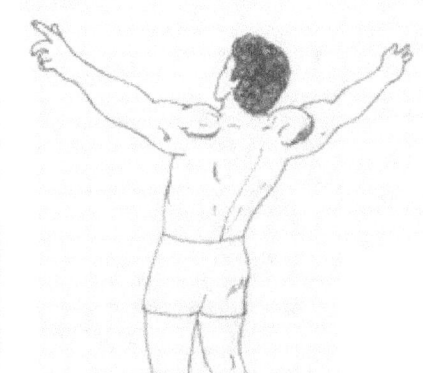

The picture above is taken from my friend Shen's webpage, and is an example of VRT exercise methods.

Stretch – The "Good morning" back stretch. From a wide stance, spread your arms up and out and back, and lean backward. Stretch your arms way out and back. Concentrate on the tension on your shoulders, feel the blood rushing into those muscle cells. Hold for 10 seconds. This exercise will also contribute to good posture.

Go here for more:

http://www.angelfire.com/ny5/shenandoah/OBB/

Sandbag Training

This item from the list is another one that may have some of you scratching your heads.

Sandbag training is not new, but it has gained some recent popularity in some training circles. Sand is cheap and versatile, conforming to its container's shape.

A bag of sand weighing 50 pounds is about $3 at your construction supply store or hardware outlet, so you can purchase plenty of resistance without breaking the budget.

As I have a page on my website dedicated to "frugal fitness" (http://christianiron.com/FrugalFitness.aspx), I love cheap tools and methods for getting stronger, and sandbags definitely fit that bill. You can put them in a backpack or a duffel bag and then put the weight on your back or lift, carry or even throw the sand-filled duffel bag. You can even fill handled laundry containers and coffee containers, etc., with sand to make your own outdoor ready weights! You can also make your own medicine balls by opening up a basketball, soccer ball or such and filling with sand and sealing with epoxy, fiberglass, or tape.

A duffel bag with well sealed plastic bags full of sand can be used to perform various exercises, and it's shifting and awkwardness actually add a challenging component that makes it superior to standard weight training movements in some regards.

You can deadlift, squat, press, row or curl the bag. Toss the bag back and forth between yourself and your training partner for a very explosive "Plyometrics" style workout.

You can perform strongman style moves like the farmers walk with buckets or bags of sand, or you can put a backpack on and jump up as high as you can out of a deep squat position for explosive leg power. Do these for repetitions for a real calorie burning inferno.

Throw a bag or two of sand in a wheelbarrow and push it up a steep hill as fast as you can, or just sprint up the hill holding the bag in front of you. Are these ideas a little too extreme for you? They are not for the faint of heart, that's for sure.

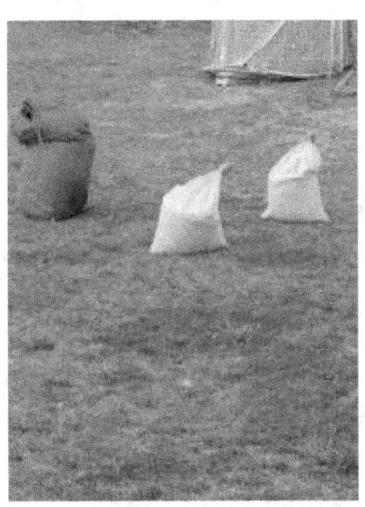

Gymnastics

While most of us think about the more formal Olympic type of exercises when they see or hear this word, it is not necessarily what I had in mind when I added it to my list.

To be sure, that type of gymnastics is a very demanding and a great source of calorie reduction.

I was thinking of a perhaps scaled down version, using small vertical and horizontal jumping, sliding and similar movements.

Some of the old time strongmen used to jump over tables and chairs as part of their shows, or just for fun and exercise.

I would not suggest starting out by trying to jump over a table;

Try a step stool, a milk crate or something like that at first.

Having some parallel bars (you can even use something like a cheap pair of saw horses in a pinch), you can walk your body across them or swing your torso back and forth akin to the real Olympic movement. The playground workout that was mentioned on the list is really a form of gymnastics, when you get down to it.

This can be another fun and rewarding, non-conventional means of getting in your exercise.

Boxing and Martial Arts

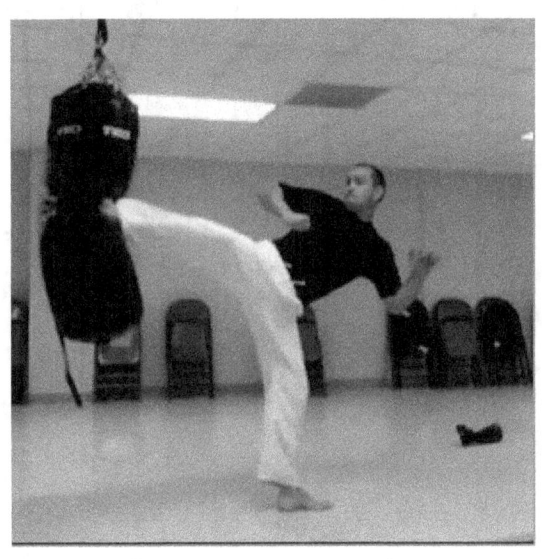

Steve Mathews
Previous interviewee at Christianiron.com
Martial arts trainer

\

You don't have to join a boxing gym or a dojo to get some good calorie melting exercise from these forms.

If you have access to a heavy bag, a speed bag, or one of those punch dummies that have become so popular, you can get a great workout by just flailing away with your arms and legs at the target.

Use over-sized gloves to add extra challenge with the added weight. You will get tired very quickly punching a bag wearing 16 ounce gloves, believe you me.

I recall back in high school when our gym teacher had us box for gym class. He provided us with 16 ounce gloves and let a couple of us go at it. Being adolescent boys, we looked forward to getting in the ring with each other so we could knock each other's block off.

In reality, after a couple of short minutes swinging those huge gloves at our opponents, we just wanted to quit and get out of the ring and catch our breath, regardless of how many blows we had dealt or received. Boxers are in good cardio condition, especially the lighter class boxers, because of the way they train. There is more to boxing than punching power. One must possess endurance, power, strength endurance and agility to be the best.

Try some boxing training in the form of an endurance building distance run, hitting the heavy bag, hitting the speed bag and jumping some rope, then toss in some strength training in the form of some standard weight movements or bodyweight, and you have quite a well rounded and challenging program.

Using Stairs

We touched on stairs in another section, but let's go into a bit more detail. There is a gentleman I routinely get emails from that has an entire exercise program built around using stairs.

You can walk or run up stairs, one step at a time, or skipping a step or two on each "rep".

You could mount each step sideways. You could perform lunges on the lower steps in a staircase. You can add weight to your body to make stair climbing more challenging, using ankle weights, the previously mentioned sandbag laden backpacks, etc.

Bounding up a set of stairs from left to right alternately on each step adds another dimension to the mix.

Stairs can be found universally, so you can use them for a quick and convenient and CHEAP workout any time.

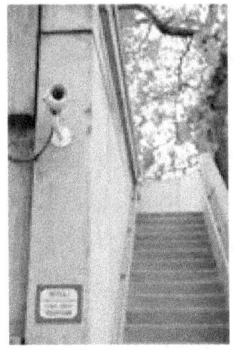

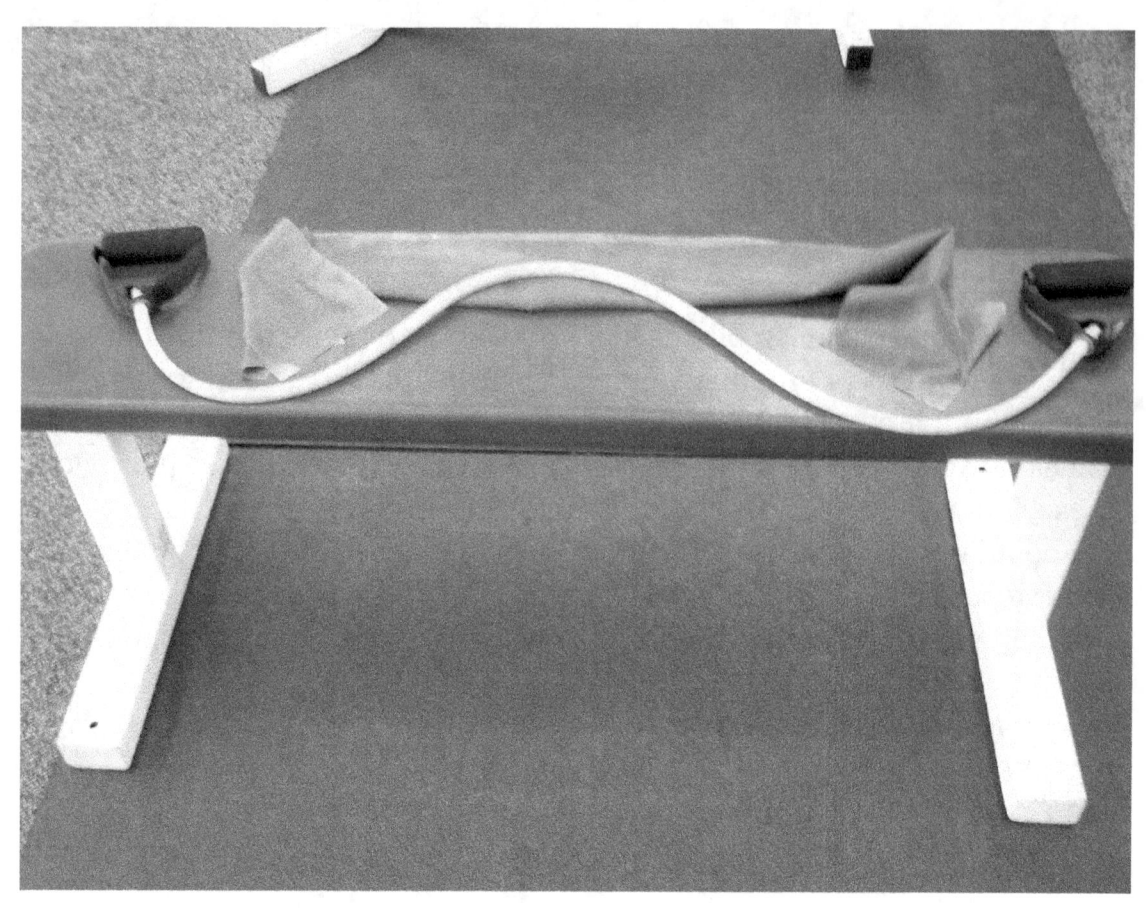

Bands& Tubes

Bands and tubes can be used to perform lots of traditional and not so traditional exercises, and they are another frugal fitness favorite.

Unlike traditional weight training equipment, they are very light and can be packed just about anywhere with ease.

Bands and tubing come in varying resistances to fit most if not all trainees' requirements. They provide resistance through an entire range of motion as opposed to weights where there is little or no resistance in certain sections of the movement. Consider for example the barbell curl. The maximum resistance is at the very bottom, and the resistance past the point where the elbow is at a 45 degree angle becomes minimal. The same movement done with an elastic tube provides *increased tension* for that same region, thus being even better than the barbell curl in that regard.

You can also hit the muscles from a wide variety of angles and positions that would be at best very tough to duplicate with weights. You can improve on many standard weight training movements by adding resistance bands to the bar, to create what is called "accommodating resistance" to work the top of the range of motion more than would be possible with just weights.

All in all, a very versatile and worthwhile type of training equipment is found in these tubes and bands.

Other methods and equipment

The list given has many ideas, but is by no means an exhaustive or all inclusive one. There are many more ideas and the imagination can come up with multiple variations and combinations of the ideas already given.

One other good piece of equipment I neglected to put on the list is trampolines, both standard sized and miniature.

Just jumping up and down on one of these is a surprisingly good workout. Mix in some callisthenic type movements while jumping and you have made a good thing that much better.

Various backyard sports such as horseshoes, badminton, bocce ball, croquet and others are fun ways to get some exercise in.

Anything that gets you moving is worthwhile and should not be written off or taken for granted.

There are a number of outdoor games that require no more equipment than a ball of some sort. When I was a lad, we played a host of vigorous games with small rubber balls we could buy for about a quarter. Wall ball, box ball, handball, step ball and wire ball are just a few that jump to mind when I think back on those days.

A couple of other things we might mention are Tai *Chi, Yoga and Pilates.* None of these is tremendous at calorie burning, but all are good forms of exercise, and are especially advocated for older folks or folks that have been sedentary for some time.

Leagues, organized sports

There are numerous sports that folks of all ages can engage in that can all provide some level of exercise. Softball, baseball, football, soccer, hockey; the list goes on.

These are all fine ways to get some fun exercise as well as gaining the other benefits that go along with being a part of a team.

Playing 1 or 2 nights a week of any of these sports is seldom enough without some additional work in other areas, however.

We must also keep in mind that stretching before, during and after these games can be very helpful in preventing injuries and staying more limber.

Staying "warm" while waiting around during periods of inactivity is strongly suggested and this will help your game and your long-term health.

Show up early to your league games if you possibly can, so that you can warm up and get some stretching in prior to game time.

You will be glad you did, I assure you.

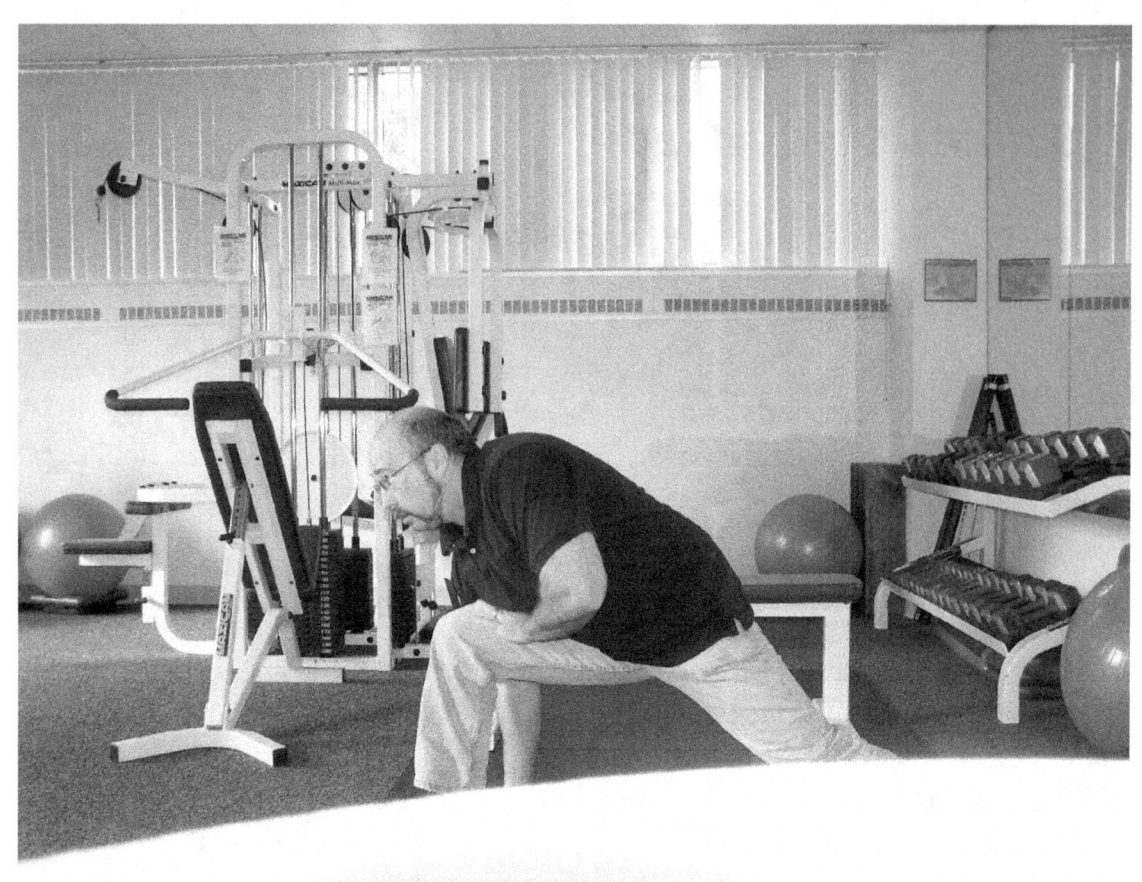

Yours truly doing some leg stretching at the gym

Chapter Eleven

The most important exercise

I made you wait until the last few pages of the book to talk about the most important exercise?!?

Well, yes, only because I thought it fit best in the **summary** section.

No, I am not talking about that top secret exercise you can perform for only 5 minutes daily to get all the benefits you ever desired.

What I am talking about is actually a mental exercise rather than a physical one.

I am referring to exercising the **will**. The will is going to be required to get you motivated and to help push you along through every phase of your new healthy lifestyle.

Yes, I said new healthy **lifestyle!**

Forget about "diets" and short lived exercise regimens that whip you into shape over night. Plan on making and keeping reasonable, doable, positive changes for the long haul.

We do not often think of it this way, but the will is something that grows stronger with exercise just like a muscle. The term "strong-willed" is often associated with stubborn people or in-subordinate children, and usually has negative connotations.

Perhaps we need to re-examine this concept a bit. Maybe being stubborn or "strong-willed" in at least some areas of life actually has some benefits.

I think you might agree that most folks who have accomplished great things in life have done so largely by being stubborn and bull-headed about getting it done, regardless of the obstacles involved.

If you really want something bad enough, you will continue to work on it and work on it until you have achieved your ultimate goal.

The "power of positive thinking" is an often used phrase, and one I am quite fond of using myself, but if this positive thinking is not matched with physical effort or "sweat equity", it will not get the job done all by itself. You can recite a mantra to the tune of "I will lose fat, I will get stronger, I will be healthier" over and over, but that alone will get you nowhere.

That kind of thinking is just conditioning the mind in a positive way to prepare it for "battle".

Make no mistake; getting in shape and staying in shape will be a battle of sorts. The more out of shape you are to begin with, the tougher the battle will be at first. But I promise you it will be worth all the effort if you stick it out. For some, eating properly or reducing calories will present the biggest challenge, while for others, getting into a regular exercise program will be the hardest part.

The key is *gradual progression.* You can't expect to go from 6000 calories a day to 2000 a day instantly, nor go from being completely sedentary to working out 3 hours per day, 6 days per week in a short time.

Even though it is possible to do something like this, and it has indeed been done, it is not even advisable to introduce such drastic changes to the body so quickly.

www.ingramcontent.com/pod-product-compliance
Lightning Source LLC
Chambersburg PA
CBHW052003280526
45793CB00005B/839